ENGAGING BLACK AND MINORITY ETHNIC GROUPS IN HEALTH RESEARCH

'Hard to Reach'? Demystifying the Misconceptions

Natalie Darko

D1612578

P

First published in Great Britain in 2023 by

Policy Press, an imprint of
Bristol University Press
University of Bristol
1-9 Old Park Hill
Bristol
BS2 8BB
UK
t: +44 (0)117 374 6645
e: bup-info@bristol.ac.uk

Details of international sales and distribution partners are available at
policy.bristoluniversitypress.co.uk

Contents

List of figures and tables   iv
Acknowledgements   v

Introduction   1

1   Concepts and misconceptions   5

2   Race, ethnicity and health inequalities   19

3   Improving research on race, ethnicity and health inequalities 37

4   The importance of intersectionality   45

5   Case study: "We are not hard to reach, you are just not   53
     reaching us!" Understanding intersectionality and the
     prevention and management of Type 2 diabetes among
     British African-Caribbean women

6   South Asian and BME migrant women's experiences   93
     of culturally tailored, women-only physical activity
     programme for improving participation, social isolation
     and wellbeing

7   Experiences of health and wellbeing during periods   107
     of fragile and uncertain citizenship among African-
     Caribbean migrant groups

Conclusion   137

References   141
Index   173

List of figures and tables

Figures

5.1   Diagrammatic map illustrating the codes and the   76
        developed themes with application of the intersectionality
        framework for one of the RE-AIM dimensions

Tables

5.1   Programme activities   63
5.2   RE-AIM framework interview guide with community   66
        participants, staff and stakeholders
5.3   Intentionality analysis template combined with   71
        RE-AIM framework
6.1   Participation data   99
7.1   Life story interview guide   116

Acknowledgements

There are many people who have kindly contributed their support to the writing of this book. I would like to say thanks to colleagues and friends at the Centre for BME Health, Leicester, and those at my new work home: The Stephen Lawrence Research Centre. I especially want to say thank you to Julian Harrison and Barbara Czyznikowska, whose expertise and passion for research with ethnic minority groups, equality, diversity, inclusion (and everything else in this field without an acronym), have been inspiring and supportive. I'd also like to say thanks to many of my other friends and colleagues working in academia and community engagement, who spend their lives listening to the voices of underrepresented ethnic minority groups and who continually remind researchers, practitioners and commissioners about the lived experiences of minority groups that are missed or ignored in research and practice.

Thank you also to Amelia Watts-Jones and Laura Vickers-Rendall and everyone else at Policy Press / Bristol University Press for allowing me to write this text and for all their support in making it an enjoyable and rapid process.

I am especially grateful to the reviewers for their support and feedback. There was so much more I wanted to include and write about that wasn't feasible here, so I'll take your recommendations forward in my future writing. I would like to give a special thanks to all the participants who took the time to participate and support this research. I only hope that change is on the horizon and that you no longer continue to be perceived as hard to reach and underrepresented!

A huge thanks to my wonderful husband, who has supported me through this entire process and in so much more – your passion for change and feedback has been wonderful. Finally, thanks to our three wonderful girls, Maya, Zadie and Leah – you are an inspiration.

Introduction

The term 'hard to reach' is not recent; it is a commonly used term and regularly applied to Black and Minority Ethnic (BME) groups in public health, health research and healthcare services. However, the concept and application to these groups is part of the problem for furthering the marginalisation and inequalities they experience in health and healthcare access.

Academics and healthcare practitioners and providers have been debating this term for some time; however, they have made little progress in advancing the term and the exclusionary practices that accompany its application. The purpose of writing this book is to illustrate how this term plays a debilitating role in othering and problematising BME people within health research and services. This is because it is often synonymised with other terms, such as 'vulnerable', 'challenging', 'marginalised', 'forgotten', 'less worthy' and 'disadvantaged' (Edge, 2013; Rockliffe et al, 2018; Sydor, 2013; Bamidele et al, 2019).

What will be considered here, is whether these groups are hard to reach – or are health researchers and health service providers and practitioners just not trying hard enough to understand their health, and the practices required to engage with these groups? Furthermore, are health services and health research practices culturally competent, and do they address issues of equality that prevent access, involvement and engagement?

The aim of this book is to also illustrate that we need to shift away from the use of the term 'hard to reach' in health services and research, because it contributes to exclusionary practices and has implications for escalating inequalities in health and healthcare access for BME groups. This is evident because BME people are still being treated differently by health service providers and health researchers, and feel unequal to White British groups (Salway et al, 2016; Race Disparity Unit, 2019a).

Furthermore, ethnic minority groups generally have poorer health than the general population, but the evidence and methods utilised to understand these health inequalities and the factors that contribute to them, are often inaccurate and inappropriate. Unfortunately, it is also commonly assumed within this field that the existence of ethnic health inequalities is due partly to these hard-to-reach groups. This is because they are presumed to be difficult to engage in healthcare and research, and their health practices or behaviours do not align with those of the majority white population, for which services and research are designed.

It is also often implied that they do not take the required health tests or screening, attend the required appointments or engage in the research – and their race, ethnicity, migrant status, behaviour and practices are perceived to be the reason for their ill health. We have witnessed this recently in the examination and management of the global COVID-19 (SARS-CoV-2) pandemic. The higher rates of incidence and deaths among BME groups has been recognised and evidenced in public health research, and by the current Conservative government (ONS, 2011; Public Health England, 2020a; Lacobucci, 2020a; Niedzwiedz et al, 2020). For example, the UK Conservative Secretary of State for Health and Social Care, Matt Hancock, recognised in June 2020, "the disproportionate way that this disease targets people … who are from black or minority ethnic backgrounds" (House of Lords, 3 June 2020).

However, the causes of this virus that lie in the wider determinants of ethnic health inequalities have been largely ignored at ministerial level and in public health discourse. Notably, the voices of BME groups and stakeholders who have provided insight into these causes, have either not been listened to or temporarily forgotten in research and public health reports (Bhopal, 2020). Furthermore, there have been problems and inaccuracies in the recording and monitoring of race and ethnicity to understand and address this condition in health research and public health practice. All of these practices need to be addressed, as they contribute to the invisibility of BME groups in health services and research, and thus there is a continued focus on these groups as being hard to reach.

The recent focus on police brutality and the killing of unarmed black African Americans, such as George Floyd, in the US in 2020, has led to a public focus on racial injustice across all aspects of society, and notably in health in the UK. These occurrences remind us that we must do more to address the inequalities that still exist in our society. Matt Hancock, the UK Secretary of State for Health and Social Care, himself recognised that: 'black lives matter … and should not be forgotten in healthcare and research and … has exposed the huge disparities in the health of our nation' (House of Lords, 3 June 2020). We need to introduce change, to give greater meaning to this statement.

As health researchers, practitioners and healthcare providers, we can do much more to understand why these disparities in health occur and how racial injustices, discrimination and other social, political and cultural practices can have an impact. The chapters in this book aim to explore some of the exclusionary practices that occur in health research and practice, and provide guidance for practitioners and researchers on how to avoid misconceptions about BME groups and how to improve practice.

Chapter 1 outlines key understandings of race and ethnicity and terms such as 'BME' and 'BAME' (Black, Asian and Minority Ethnic) and how they are applied in this text. It then focuses on outlining the term 'hard to reach' and its assignment to BME populations in health services and research (Lamb et al, 2012; Liljas et al, 2017; Rockliffe et al, 2018; Liljas et al, 2019). Here a historical account of the terms and of the challenges faced when doing inclusive research is discussed. This chapter aligns to existing research in this field, which acknowledges that BME people are still being treated differently by service providers and feel unequal to White British groups (Salway et al, 2016; Race Disparity Unit, 2019a). The implications of current exclusionary practices in research are discussed. Importantly, the chapter provides guidance for practitioners and researchers on how to apply the discussed terms to their own practice.

Chapter 2 outlines understanding of the relationship between race, ethnicity and health (Karlsen et al, 2012; Kumar and Diaz, 2019). An exploration of the current research that details health outcomes and health-related practices of BME people in the UK is given (Race Disparity Unit, 2019b; Millan and Smith, 2019).

In Chapter 3, it is acknowledged that there are differences in healthcare outcomes by ethnicity and that this is hampered by poor quality data. Thus, improvements need to be made to improve the visibility of BME groups and the methods utilised to research them (Bhopal, 1997, 2007). It is also argued that by improving the equality and cultural competency of health researchers, we can also improve the visibility of diverse BME groups in health research and practice.

Chapter 4 focuses on intersectionality, and discusses why it is important for the delivery of health interventions for BME groups. In recognition of recent research on intersectionality, additional dimensions of difference for ethnic minority people are discussed here (Reimer-Kirkham and Sharma, 2011; Mwangi and Constance-Huggins, 2017). Following a brief exploration of some of the current health interventions and studies that employ, or argue for, an intersectional approach, it is argued that few in the UK facilitate a focus on this approach and its impact on health and access to healthcare interventions for BME people (Tomalin et al, 2019).

This sets the context for Chapter 5, in which a research case study is presented about why intersectionality theory is important for addressing misconceptions about African–Caribbean women as being hard to reach in health intervention delivery. Recommendations are given to improve the development of health interventions by involving British African–Caribbean women in the design and provision of culturally tailored interventions in their communities, and by applying intersectionality theory and methodological frameworks.

Chapter 6 focuses on the delivery and evaluation of a community-based programme designed to improve physical activity, social isolation and wellbeing among South Asian and BME migrant women living in areas of high economic deprivation. The chapter provides an accessible insight into the aims, objectives, methods and findings of the study. It provides recommendations on how researchers and service providers can deliver culturally tailored, community-based health interventions. It demonstrates how to mitigate misconceptions about South Asian and BME migrant women being hard to reach and difficult to engage in physical activity health interventions.

Chapter 7 provides an insight into how participants of African–Caribbean heritage have experienced their health, wellbeing and healthcare access since their arrival to the UK and during periods of fragile and uncertain citizenship. This includes exploration of the risks for the wellbeing of existing residents whose migrant status has become uncertain. Life storytelling methods are utilised, to produce bibliographic accounts of the participants who moved to the UK at any time from the 1940s to the present day, or whose immediate family did so. The chapter draws attention to the ways in which future research can be delivered in collaboration with BME migrants, to understand their migration journeys and its impact on health.

1

Concepts and misconceptions

Terms such as 'race', 'ethnicity', 'BME' (Black and Minority Ethnic) and 'BAME' (Black, Asian and Minority Ethnic) are commonly used in health practice and research. However, understanding of the terms varies and they are commonly misunderstood. This chapter provides a brief outline of the meanings frequently used for these terms and how they are applied in this text.

Attention then focuses on the concept of 'hard to reach' and its assignment to BME populations who do not engage in health services and research (Lamb et al, 2012; Liljas et al, 2017; Rockliffe et al, 2018; Liljas et al, 2019). The reasons why BME people are conceptualised in this way in health services and research are also discussed. It is recognised that academics and practitioners have been debating these issues for some time, but have made little progress in advancing the term and the exclusionary practices that accompany its application. Reflecting on when and why this has occurred, is an important starting point for introducing this text. Therefore, a historical account of the concept of 'hard to reach' is provided and the challenges faced when doing inclusive research are discussed.

The final section of this chapter highlights the problems of utilising this term. Specifically, it is argued that the term 'hard to reach' plays a debilitating role in 'othering' BME people within health services, as it is often synonymised with other terms such as: 'vulnerable', 'problematic', 'marginalised', 'forgotten', 'less worthy' and 'disadvantaged' (Edge, 2013; Rockliffe et al, 2018; Sydor, 2013; Bamidele et al, 2019).

This chapter aligns to existing research in this field, which acknowledges that BME people are still being treated differently by service providers and feel unequal to White British groups (Salway et al, 2016; Race Disparity Unit, 2019a). The implications of current exclusionary practices in research are discussed.

Key concepts

When completing research or working with different groups of people, it is essential that key concepts regarding their identity are understood.

Misconceptions of these concepts can impact significantly on how the research or a programme of work is conducted and how the participants engage with the process.

Race and ethnicity are concepts that refer to features or characteristics of a person's identity that allow us to differentiate between people and/or groups (Kumar and Diaz, 2019). These concepts are often intertwined or misunderstood by researchers and practitioners, and they can be used inappropriately to identify, classify and categorise individuals and groups. The concepts of BME (Black and Minority Ethnic) or BAME (Black, Asian and Minority Ethnic) can add to this confusion, as they include a combination of one's race and ethnicity (Johnson et al, 2019). To improve practice and our engagement with these different groups, it is useful to outline key understandings of race and ethnicity, BME/BAME, 'hard to reach' and their historical origins.

Conceptualising race and the historical context

'Race' is currently understood in health research and applied practice as a biological category that refers to one's skin colour (Malik, 1996; Mason, 2000). However, it is a contentious term that has been informed historically by biological determinism and scientific racism that aligns race to individual worth.

From as early as the 19th century, biological determinists assumed that human behaviour was directly controlled by an individual's component of their physiology, that being their racial identity (Malik, 1996). Biological determinists, such as Charles Darwin (1859), believed that environmental factors had no influence on a person's innate properties such as race. They were perceived to be based on biology and were the key to understanding social identities and problems (Taylor, 1981).

This stood in opposition to the notion of race as being socially constructed ('constructivism'). At this time, ethnologists and physical anthropologists ranked people by their race and differential worth, utilising physical measurements of the body, the skull size and the brain to inform this. Criminologist Cesare Lombroso and physician Paul Broca asserted that those with black skin were different and less superior to white non-European people (Broca, 1864; Lombroso et al, 2006; LaPointe, 2021). In contrast, those with white skin were classed as being positioned within the upper hierarchies of society. It is at this time and during the second half of the 19th century that biological determinism began to intersect with scientific racism, in which the white race was classified as superior, thus justifying white supremacy, slavery and segregation in Britain and beyond. Biological sciences and the work of Broca and Lombroso were used, by some, to inform and uphold key arguments of racial difference and racial prejudice to promote scientific racism (La Pointe, 2012). Key political thinkers and academics, such as Benjamin Kidd and Karl Pearson, also drew on the basis of Darwin's determinist ideas to support colonialism and territorial expansion. Through social Darwinism, oppression of the inferior races was seen by them as being essential to the political and economic survival of Britain at that time (Dennis, 1995).

The concept of race at this time was also informed by the movement of eugenics and its naturalist founder Francis Galton (1883). Unlike social Darwinism, eugenicists wanted to modify and enhance the existing white race, to ensure that the less inferior races were unable to expand. This led to intelligence testing, in which those with lower levels of intelligence (IQ) were perceived to be responsible for social problems and thus required sterilisation. This approach spread globally, particularly in the United States (US) and in Germany. Notably, a key proponent of this movement included Adolf Hitler, who passed a law in 1933 that sought to prevent the spread of further generations by provision of compulsory sterilisation. In the US, Gabriel (1940) and Arthur Jensen (1869) followed Galton's (1883) tradition, by claiming that black African Americans were less intelligent than their white counterparts and should be subject to sterilisation, along with criminals and the insane. His work was utilised by those who opposed desegregation at that time (Dennis, 1995). While race at this time was perceived as biological, the political context in which race was conceptualised played an inherent part. It was utilised as an opportunity to maintain superiority of the white majority race and to subjugate the inferior.

During the 19th century, we saw a shift in the perception of race as being aligned to one's behaviour and worth. The belief in the validity of race as a biological concept was undermined, as cultural anthropologists discovered that the typologies of particular races were inconsistent. They found that: 'numerous distinct populations did not conform to the accepted categories and any classifications became hopelessly entangled in themes of ethnicity and nationality' (Barkan, 1992: 3). Further critiques of biological determinism and scientific racism questioned these methods and claims regarding the innate differences between races (Gould, 1980). Academics and critical thinkers then began discriminating between fact and opinion and the political discourses of race at that time.

The concept of race was brought into doubt by social reformers and social scientists, who challenged the authority of scientific racism and its link to the oppression of minority races (Taylor, 1981). W.E.B. Du Bois

(1968) was one of the key social reformists who opposed the concept of race as a determining factor in human affairs. He challenged scientific racism, social Darwinism, the eugenics movement, and psychologists' measurement of intelligence, for the weak methodologies and its biased researchers (Taylor, 1981). Importantly, he presented evidence that refuted claims of insanity, criminality and low intelligence among black African Americans (Du Bois, 1968). Du Bois offered the opportunity for activists, social scientists and civil rights leaders to question the concept of race and its claimed link to biology. In key works he noted the arbitrariness of the concept of race and the important impact that historical and social phenomena have on its definition and function (Du Bois, 1968). He argued for the substitution of the biological definition of race to a socio-historical one that recognises how the concept of race is informed by the social and historical factors that constitute its meaning. Its meaning is constitutively constructed in the history, traditions, practices and language of that race at that time. The influence of social scientists such as Du Bois, and the shift toward social constructivism, informed the new concept of 'ethnicity' and its distinction from race.

Ethnicity

The term 'ethnicity' or 'ethnic' has been utilised from as early as 750 BC by the Greeks. Its meaning in Greek biblical text refers to non-Christian or non-Jewish populations, and the adjective *ethnikos* is employed to describe them as 'pagan', 'heathen' or 'barbarian' (Fenton, 2003; Gabbart, 2006).

The contemporary academic usage of the term 'ethnic' began in the early 19th century, and was inspired by opponents of scientific racism, social Darwinism and eugenics, who opposed the interchangeable use of race, nation, class and ethnicity (Gabbart, 2006). Currently, common general conceptions of ethnicity recognise that ethnicity refers to one's cultural and social identity and difference, and that race in contrast is a biological and genetic referent (Mulholland and Dyson, 2001).

Different approaches to the meaning of ethnicity

However, there have been varying approaches to the meaning of ethnicity in academic research. These include primordialism, perennialism, modernism, instrumentalism and constructivism.

Primordialists argue that ethnicity has existed throughout human history and that modern ethnic groups have historical roots in the past. Ethnicity is closely aligned to the idea of nation and its inherent meaning. For them, membership of an ethnic group is acquired through one's birth and nurtured by one's family. Once ethnicity is constructed, it becomes fixed as a single identity with multiple dimensions (Geertz, 1973; Van Evera, 1981, 2001).

Perennialists argue that the concept of ethnicity is a stable feature of social organisations that has existed at all times. However, ethnic groups are perceived to be short-lived, before the ethnic boundaries realign in new patterns.

Modernists attributed the importance of ethnicity to the rise of the nation state. Instrumentalists differ, in that they argue that the meaning of ethnicity lies in individual autonomy, where the individual can choose between different identities as they see fit.

Like the instrumentalist conceptions, social constructivists perceive ethnicity as being socially constructed. However, this is achieved continuously through social interaction, by both elites and ordinary people, as opposed to just the individual themselves. This approach differs to primordialism and perennialism, as ethnic groups are perceived as products of social interaction, preserved only in so far as they are maintained as valid social constructs in societies (Chandra, 2001; Chandra and Wilkinson, 2008). Furthermore, they differ to primodialists, as constructivists assume that multiple ethnic identities exist, as opposed to a single ethnic identity (Bayar, 2010).

Despite the varying definitions of ethnicity, attempts have been made to create a more conceptual synthesis, with many adopting recognition of its socially constructed nature (Du Bois, 1968; Chandra, 2001; Eriksen, 2002; Chandra and Wilkinson, 2008; Johnson et al, 2019).

What is ethnicity?

Like 'race', the term 'ethnicity' and its meaning have, over time, been difficult to describe (Craig and Atkin, 2012). However, in academic research, 'ethnicity' is a term that often describes shared culture – the practices, values and beliefs of a group. This might include shared language, religion, descent and traditions, among other commonalities (Van den Berghe, 1981). An ethnic group is a collection of people or a social group whose members identify with each other through a common heritage, consisting of a common culture that may also include a shared language or dialect. The group's ethos or ideology may also stress common ancestry, descent, diet, religion or race. Johnson et al (2019: 86) argue that it is important to recognise that 'all people have an ethnicity — *not only minorities*'. This is often a common misconception in health practice and research: *ethnicity is often perceived as only belonging to BME groups.* What should be recognised is that there are cultural practices embedded in ethnicity for *all* groups, and these changes are dependent on social interaction. Therefore, ethnicity is transitory and subject to change.

From a constructivist perspective, the features of ethnicity are also socially constructed. In this respect, it is easy to see how ethnicity differs to race, because as discussed earlier, ethnicity refers to one's cultural and social identity [that is dependent on social interaction and change] ... whereas race is perceived as a biological referent (Mulholland and Dyson, 2001) that is more static. There are also opposing positions, which argue that race is also a social construct, similar to a person's ethnicity or ethnic group (Bhavnani et al, 2005; Craig et al, 2012; Johnson et al, 2019).

Despite the more common general conception of ethnicity and its distinction from race as a biological referent, race classifications are combined with ethnic identity in health and medical practice to label ethnic groups (Bhopal and Donaldson, 1998; Comstock and Castillo, 2004; Bhopal, 2007). Labels such as Asian, South Asian and black-African, black British, and mixed – black-African are commonly referred to as a person's 'ethnic group' in the UK, and utilised in health practice as diagnosis and treatment of disease (Bhopal, 2007).

For example, NHS monitoring records commonly sort individuals into one of approximately 20 ethnic categories. These are informed by the categories utilised by the Office for National Statistics (ONS) and the Census that encapsulate what is commonly perceived as the multidimensional nature of ethnicity. Some of the criteria used by the ONS to identify an ethnic minority group include: nationality, country of birth, language, religion, national or geographical origin, and skin colour. However, as we can see, this definition of ethnicity includes both race and ethnicity. The NHS data dictionary also encompasses a similar approach, because the ethnic code category utilises both racial identifiers (for example black) and ethnicity features. Although this practice has been critiqued (Sheldon and Parker, 1992; Bhopal, 2007), this still continues in research and healthcare practice.

This is compounded by use of the terms 'Black and Minority Ethnic' (BME) or 'Black, Asian and Minority Ethnic' (BAME) to refer to 'ethnic minorities'. These terms conflate race and ethnicity (this is discussed later). The problem in adopting this definition of ethnicity, is that researchers or practitioners often fail to differentiate between race and ethnicity. Furthermore, some can erroneously attribute health disparities to racial and ethnic group differences, and fail to adequately study and understand the actual underlying causes of the disparities.

So, what do the terms BME and BAME mean, where did these terms originate, and should we use them in health research and related practice?

Black and Minority Ethnic (BME) and Black, Asian and Minority Ethnic (BAME)

Black and Minority Ethnic (BME) or Black, Asian and Minority Ethnic (BAME) is the terminology commonly used in the UK to describe people of non-white descent. As discussed earlier, this terminology combines both a person's race and ethnicity. This terminology has sparked controversy for a number of years, because of this inclusion. This has led to further confusion of those who do not understand the distinction between these features of identity. This is not helped by use of the term 'race', which includes ethnicity or features commonly understood as relating to a person's ethnicity or background.

Notably, the Equality Act 2010 refers to 'the protected characteristic of race as a group of people defined by their race, colour and nationality (including citizenship) ethnic or national origins' (Equality Act, 2010; Human Rights and Equality Commission, 2020). Critics of the terms advocate for the use of 'ethnic minorities' as opposed to BME or BAME (Modood, 1994; Johnson et al, 2019). Furthermore, the current COVID-19 pandemic has drawn greater attention to the problems of using these terms, when trying to understand factors affecting the impact of COVID-19 on different racial groups. However, before discussing recommendations for changes to their use, it is important to understand the history of the terms BME and BAME and the current problems with their use.

The term 'BME' has its origins in the idea of 'political blackness', a term used by many in the anti-racist movement during the 1970s and 1980s in the UK (Andrews, 2016). People from different racial groups and ethnic backgrounds in the UK banded together to oppose the universal term 'black' to create an anti-racist solidarity and fight back against discrimination and violence (Narayan, 2019). Different groups worked to transform the racist victimisation of African, African-Caribbean and South Asian communities, and led campaigns for racial justice and social change (Ambikaipaker, 2018). However, since this period, activists have argued that use of this term is problematic, because of the inclusion of the term 'black'. In particular, Modood (1994) argues that the term is all encompassing, as it implies that all non-white groups are a homogeneous group and are not being treated accordingly. He also argues that the term is harmful for British Asians,

11

because it gives undue prominence to Black African and African-Caribbean people.

Since this period, adaptions of the term have been made to address this, leading to the inclusion of the term 'Black, Asian and Minority Ethnic (BAME)'. While this addresses the concerns raised by Asian activists, this arguably now singles out specific ethnic groups and can be divisive and exclusionary. For example, if we consider white invisible minorities, such as those who identify as Gypsy, Roma and Travellers, they can become disguised and forgotten within this term, because of their white racial categorisation. Yet: 'Gypsies and some Traveller ethnicities have been recognised in law as being ethnic groups protected against discrimination by the Equality Act 2010' and classified as BME within ethnicity monitoring (Cromarty, 2019: 4). The terms 'BME' or 'BAME' therefore also involve white ethnic minority groups. In the British context – and applied to Census categories – these terms refer to any ethnic grouping apart from majority white British.

If we adopt these terms BAME or BME without further education on their meaning in the respective fields, it can potentially lead some researchers and practitioners to treat *all* ethnic groups homogeneously, without recognition of the differences in both race and ethnicity. This can mask inequalities between the various ethnic groups. Furthermore, it can generally be perceived that these terms refer only to non-white people, which does not consider white minority ethnic groups.

As discussed earlier, Johnson et al (2019) also quite rightly recognise that we all have an ethnicity, and terms such as BAME/BME encourage the assumption that ethnicity is only applicable to non-white ethnic minority groups. They too argue that this term is an illogical and derogatory acronym. In their glossary for the first World Congress on Migration, Ethnicity, Race and Health, Johnson et al (2019) argue that the acronym 'BAME/BME standing for Black, Asian and Minority Ethnic or Black and Minority Ethnic is used as a shorthand for groups excluded or disadvantaged by racism and xenophobia' – thus, recommending against its use.

The debate about which term or terms we should use, if any, is more than likely to continue for some time. However, it is unlikely that a conceptual synthesis will be agreed, given the various competing political, academic and clinical positions. What can be recommended is that those using the terms 'BME' or 'BAME' in health practice and health-related research should ensure that they understand their meaning, and potentially consult with minority groups from different racial and ethnic backgrounds to ask them what term or terms they would like to be utilised. Furthermore, when utilising the term in publications, guidance, policy and practice, writers and practitioners should spell out clearly who they include in every ethnic group label, to avoid broad use of the term 'BME/BAME'. Opportunities for self-identification should also be considered, where feasible, and if the term/s are required to be changed, then researchers and practitioners should avoid them.

In this book, the terms 'BME' and 'ethnic minority groups' are used to refer to people of minority ethnic backgrounds and racial groups in the British context. This includes any ethnic grouping apart from majority White British.

Hard to reach

The term 'hard to reach' is commonly utilised across all sectors of society. Yet it is regularly used by the National Health Service (NHS) and the Department of Health when discussing or seeking to address inequalities in health and health provision. Notably, the NHS Plan and National Service Framework in 2002 acknowledge that certain groups are marginalised from services and are therefore 'harder to reach' for health providers whose goal is to provide appropriate and equitable healthcare for all (Department of Health, 2002). Furthermore, the NHS (2016) *Bite-Size Guide to Diverse and Inclusive Participation* refers to improving inclusivity by 'connecting with those who we find hardest to reach'. More recently, Lord Bethell, Conservative Parliamentary Under-Secretary for the Department of Health and Social Care, used the term in the House of Commons on 2 June 2020 to refer to vulnerable BME groups. He identified these groups as taking the fewest number of COVID-19 (SARS-CoV-2) tests, despite them being at a higher risk. He aimed to improve testing in these groups by 'ensur[ing] that … marketing messages are focused on the right communities' (House of Lords Covid-19 Response, 2020).

While the term 'hard to reach' is commonly used, it is an ambiguous and contested term, because there are various definitions and it is often applied in different contexts (Cook, 2002). However, it is most frequently applied to people who are members of ethnic minority groups, homeless people, asylum seekers, refugees, drug users and those who are perceived as inaccessible or less accessible than a majority group, often the White British group (Shaghaghi et al, 2011). This includes any ethnic grouping apart from majority White British.

Health researchers and healthcare practitioners describe these groups, who are perceived to be difficult to reach or to involve in research or public health programmes (Fanzana and Srunv, 2001; Hoppitt, 2012;

Liljas et al, 2017; Rockliffe et al, 2018; Liljas et al, 2019). However, the term has negative connotations for those targeted, as it suggests that they are somehow more difficult to communicate with than other audiences. Furthermore, its use is often accompanied by preconceptions that can lead to depicting these audiences as the 'other' – powerless, apathetic, vulnerable, marginalised, problematic, and less worthy within health services and health-related research (Edge, 2013; Sydor, 2018; Bamidele et al, 2019).

What should be considered, is whether these groups are hard to reach – or are researchers and service providers just not trying hard enough to understand the practices required to engage with these groups? With this in mind, it is important to consider whether health services and health research practices are culturally competent, and do they address issues of equality that prevent access, involvement and engagement? If this is the case, should we consider an alternative term, such as 'underserved', 'seldom heard', 'hidden populations' or 'hard to hear' (Atkinson and Flint, 2001). The NHS *Five-Year Forward View* (2014) refers to 'underserved groups' as opposed to 'hard to reach'; however, other NHS guidance and policy continues to utilise the term 'hard to reach' when referring to minority groups from different racial groups and ethnic backgrounds. These new terms imply that these groups are easily accessible, but they may lack the confidence or resources (financial, knowledge or skills) to engage in a particular project or in healthcare. Furthermore, these terms can help to raise concerns about the ability of the health services to provide care for all and about the techniques used by researchers to address the equality and equity of access.

Origins of the term 'hard to reach'

Before we consider this and look at recommendations for practice, a historical account of the term 'hard to reach' – and its assignment to BME or ethnic minority populations in health services and research – is given here. By doing this, we can perhaps understand why BME people are conceptualised in this way, and discuss the problems that can arise when doing inclusive research.

The origins of the term 'hard to reach' in health services can be traced back to marketing strategies within the field of health promotion in the 1980s (Beder, 1980; Walsh et al, 1993). The pejorative use of the term stems from its use in a 2004 Home Office Report, in which 'minority groups' are typified alongside the 'service resistant' who are unwilling to engage with service providers (Doherty et al, 2004).

But why have ethnic minority groups been conceptualised in this way in health services? Some argue that the term serves to stigmatise minority groups and maintain their marginalisation from mainstream society (Freimuth and Mettger, 1990; Tritter and Lester, 2007). It has also been suggested that the term is utilised to raise awareness of the threat that these groups can pose to the public health agenda and emphasise the need to change their behaviour and engage. By inferring that there is an unwillingness of these groups to engage or to 'be reached', preconceptions arise that these groups are fatalistic, and an accompanying sense of apathy impacts on *their* health, healthcare access and engagement in health research (Freimuth and Mettger, 1990). Researchers adopting this approach will focus more on what *can be done to* engage with and *encourage these groups* to access preventative healthcare services, rather than understanding the inequalities that may impact on their access (Rockliffe et al, 2018). This plays a part in attaching responsibility of health or engagement to the individual, in which it is the duty of that person to change their behaviour or reduce their risk of preventable disease, rather than attributing fault in the healthcare system or research practice (Freimuth and Mettger, 1990). This approach shifts attention away from the barriers that ethnic minorities face in accessing services and research and the inequalities that may be influential to this. It does not tell us the whole story about the problem, and only acknowledges it in the context of providing a service to a majority white group (Flanagan and Hancock, 2010). It also defines the problem as one within the group itself, and not within the researcher's or providers' approach to them.

When classifying people as being hard to reach, researchers can potentially face problems in doing inclusive research. Notably, researchers indirectly imply a homogeneity within groups that does not exist. Certain groups, such as BME older people (Liljas et al, 2017, 2019) are perceived as a homogeneous group that are all hard to reach. However, there is much diversity within and between these groups (Freimuth and Mettger, 1990; Tritter and Lester, 2007). Individuals who fall within this category do not form a standardised group. Specific sub-groups within this category may access each individual service or research study differently, and the factors that impact on this vary widely (Rockliffe et al, 2018). For example, people from different ethnic backgrounds and racial groups such as African American, African-Caribbean, African, Vietnamese, Spanish, Cantonese-speaking, Punjabi-speaking, Asian, black, and mixed Other can be grouped together as a hard-to-reach BME groups – thus implying that the practices needed for all BME groups are relatively similar.

Yet, as discussed earlier, there are differences between ethnicities, and between ethnic and racial groups, that must be acknowledged, and the strategies and recommendations for one sub-group will differ to another with a different ethnic background. We should consider that despite similarities in categorisation of BME identity, the one-size approach does not fit all (Lamb et al, 2012; Bamidele et al, 2019).

The implications of taking this approach and implying homogeneity are significant, because it can lead to exclusionary practice. If we consider the requirements of the Equality Act 2020, which tackles disadvantage and discrimination, and of equality practice measures such as equality impact assessments, then recommendations can be given by researchers that promote further exclusionary practices and decision-making processes that are unfair and which maintain barriers to participation for protected groups (Equality and Human Rights Commission, 2020).

Notably, if different ethnic groups are identified as having similar needs or facilitators to encourage their participation in research, have the needs of the individual of each 'race' been met? The Equality Act 2010 states that it is against the law if someone discriminates against you or treats you differently because they think you belong to a certain racial group even though you don't. Misconceptions about the strategies employed for one racial group could be confused and applied to another group, on assumption that this person belongs to that group. This could lead to discrimination by perception of race.

It is therefore important that researchers are cautious when applying the term 'hard to reach' to all groups from different racial groups and ethnic backgrounds. Or, as discussed earlier, they should move away from employing this term and consider alternatives, such as 'seldom heard' or 'underserved'.

Conclusion

This chapter has highlighted that we need to think differently about the terms we employ, when doing inclusive practice in health and health-related research. The terms and typologies we use to identify and classify people from different ethnic backgrounds and racial groups can impact on how these groups are understood and interpreted by others.

It is vital that researchers understand the meanings of these core terms and, most importantly, the distinction between race and ethnicity. Terms such as BME or BAME lead to the conflation of the meaning of race and ethnicity, and do not help to educate people about the difference between a person's race and their ethnicity. This also leads to further marginalisation.

As we have seen, all of these terms can be utilised by dominant and majority groups to legitimise hierarchies, and maintain segregation, marginalisation and discrimination toward minorities. This is important, because research in this field acknowledges that people from different ethnic backgrounds and racial groups are still being treated differently by service providers and feel unequal to White British groups (Salway et al, 2016; Race Disparity Unit, 2019a). Furthermore, perceived discrimination among ethnic minority groups is relatively high in healthcare settings and can lead to them forgoing healthcare (Rivenbark and Ichou, 2020).

In light of this, we need to be more cautious about the practices we utilise in both healthcare and research practice that can exacerbate perceptions of discrimination and distrust among minority groups. The lack of inclusionary practice can potentially increase health disparities among minority groups and encourage them to become hard to reach.

2

Race, ethnicity and health inequalities

Health inequalities are a growing concern in the UK. However, as the ethnic and racial diversity of the population is continuing to increase, ethnic health inequalities are rising rapidly. This chapter explores some of the key ethnic health inequalities in the UK. It begins by briefly outlining understandings of the relationship between race, ethnicity and health, to allow for an explicit consideration of ethnicity and race within health inequalities (Karlsen et al, 2012; Kumar and Diaz, 2019).

The chapter also briefly explores some of the current research data on the health outcomes and health-related practices of Black and Minority Ethnic (BME) people in the UK, to draw attention to ethnic health inequalities (Race Disparity Unit, 2019b; Millan and Smith, 2019). (As discussed in Chapter 1, the terms 'BME' and 'ethnic minority groups' used in this book refer to people of minority ethnic backgrounds and racial groups in the British context. This includes any ethnic grouping apart from majority White British.)

Central health outcomes and health-related practices are examined, including cardiovascular disease and health-related risk factors, mental health, and COVID-19 (SARS-CoV-2). This chapter also questions why ethnic health inequalities are occurring in the UK, by considering what factors influence health outcomes.

What is the relationship between race, ethnicity and health?

There is a plethora of evidence highlighting that people from BME groups experience poorer health than other groups in the UK (Race Disparity Unit, 2019b; Millan and Smith, 2019). These disparities are commonly understood as ethnic health inequalities in the UK, and often refer to differences in health status between different ethnic minority groups that are unfair and avoidable (Public Health England, 2020).

In recent years, public health and health research have witnessed a growing interest in ethnic health inequalities (Kumar and Diaz, 2019).

The recognition of these in public health has been informed by key pieces of research evidence. Notably, large-scale surveys – such as the Fourth National Survey of BME groups (Nazroo, 1997), the Health Survey for England health of ethnic minorities study in 2004 (Sproston and Mindell, 2006), and the 2011 Census (Office for National Statistics, 2011) – have indicated that BME groups as a whole are more likely to report ill health, and that ill health among BME people starts at a younger age than in the White British groups.

While these surveys identified variations in health across ethnic groups, core overlapping factors are identifiable. Key findings show that certain BME groups experienced worse health than others. Notably, Pakistani, Bangladeshi, black African-Caribbean and White Gypsy or Irish Traveller people reported the poorest health. Furthermore, patterns of ethnic health inequalities in health vary from one health condition to the next. For example, some BME groups (such as Bangladeshi, Pakistani Indian and black African-Caribbean groups) tend to have higher rates of cardiovascular disease and diabetes than White British people (Nazroo, 1997), but lower rates of many cancers (Sproston and Mindell, 2006). African-Caribbean groups also had higher rates of mental health conditions.

Differences in gender have also been identified. For example, Bangladeshi and African-Caribbean men have the highest rates of cardiovascular disease compared to women; yet women from certain BME groups (Bangladeshi women) also have higher rates of diabetes compared with women in the general population. For example, the Health Survey for England (HMO Health and Safety Executive, 2004) reports that 'doctor-diagnosed diabetes is more than five times as likely among Pakistani women, at least three times as likely in Bangladeshi and Black Caribbean women, and two-and-a-half times as likely in Indian women compared with women in the general population' (Sproston and Mindell, 2006: 7). Furthermore, White Gypsy or Irish Traveller men are almost twice as likely to have a long-term illness than White British men.

Health among children was also examined, with figures indicating that obesity levels among ethnic groups were relatively high. Notably, black African boys were more likely to be obese than boys in the general population, and levels of obesity rose for black Caribbean and Bangladeshi boys from 1999. Inequalities in socioeconomic position were also highlighted as being highly influential to ill health in ethnic minority groups: those located in lower socioeconomic positions faced poorer health outcomes.

With the exception of the Public Health England (2020a) report on COVID-19 and Office for National Statistics COVID-19 surveys on

BME groups, there have been minimal large-scale national surveys since 2011 that have focused solely on the health of BME groups (Karlsen et al, 2012; Public Health England, 2018). The Cabinet Office's Race Disparity Unit does produce figures via the *Ethnicity, Facts and Figures* website that provide an insight into some of the differences in health (physical and mental) among ethnic groups. However, at the time of writing, there are only a sample of health conditions that are reported, such as health-related quality of life for people over 65 years of age, mental health conditions, early cancer diagnosis, and HIV infection with late diagnosis (Race Disparity Unit, 2019b). Academic research studies have also examined differences in health between ethnic groups and have found that people from ethnic minority backgrounds continue to be worst affected by poor health since 2011. Here we can look at some of these central disparities in the latest data.

Differences in health outcomes and health-related risk factors

In the large-scale surveys discussed earlier, it was evident that cardiovascular disease and health-related risk factors were higher among some ethnic minority groups. What is interesting in recent data across the surveys and key research, is that poor health among ethnic minority groups is still relatively higher than that of the general population. Thus, ethnic health inequalities still persist.

For example, a Public Health England (2018a) report entitled *Health Inequalities: Reducing ethnic inequalities, guidance to support local and national action on ethnic inequalities in health*, reported poorer health among certain ethnic minority groups. Specifically, those identifying as Gypsy or Irish Traveller, and to a lesser extent those identifying as Bangladeshi, Pakistani or Irish, have poor health across a range of indicators (Public Health England, 2018a). Furthermore, rates of infant mortality are highest among Pakistani groups, along with Pakistani, black African-Caribbean and black African groups. The latter groups, coupled into a black aggregated category within Hospital Episode Statistics and the Adult Psychiatric Morbidity Survey, also have higher levels of poor health. Notably, black groups have the highest rates of obesity, and black men have higher rates of prostate cancer and psychotic disorders than men in other ethnic groups in this report.

There are ethnic health inequalities across various health outcomes to be examined in academic research, but unfortunately there is not sufficient space to examine all of these here. Before briefly examining a few of those that have been reported more extensively, it is important to note here that the extent of the difference in health varies across health conditions and ethnic groups, so the information that follows is just a general snapshot of some of the recent research (Chouhan and Nazroo, 2020).

Cardiovascular disease and health-related risk factors

Research shows that BME groups in the UK have a higher burden of cardiovascular disease (George et al, 2017) and higher rates of Type 2 diabetes, hypertension, obesity and kidney disease than their white counterparts. For example, people of South Asian backgrounds have higher rates of cardiovascular disease than white British groups (George et al, 2017) and the prevalence of cardiovascular disease is highest in Indian, Pakistani and men (British Heart Foundation, 2010). Furthermore, the risk of stroke is higher among South Asian, black African and black African-Caribbean people (Wolfe et al, 2002; Agyemang et al, 2012; Khunti et al, 2013; Chouhan and Nazroo, 2020) compared to the majority population. There are further differences in the types of cardiovascular disease conditions presented by ethnic groups of South Asian, African, and African-Caribbean descent. These are explored in more detail in George et al (2017) and, critically, by Bhopal (2019).

Research suggests that the prevalence of Type 2 diabetes is disturbingly high among BME groups in the UK; approximately three to six times higher than in the white British population (Goff, 2019; Chouhan and Nazroo, 2020). Furthermore, the onset of Type 2 diabetes occurs much earlier for a greater proportion of ethnic minority groups, some 10–12 years younger, with a significant proportion of cases being diagnosed before the age of 40 years (Paul et al, 2017). Particular ethnic minority groups have an increased risk of developing the condition; notably, research suggests that 50% of people of South Asian, African, and African-Caribbean descent will develop diabetes by the age of 80 (Tillin et al, 2010). Furthermore, people of South Asian, African and African-Caribbean groups have been identified as being between three to six times more likely to experience Type 2 diabetes than other groups (Department of Health, 2001; Riste et al, 2001; Farmaki et al, 2020). Intergenerational differences have been identified, indicating that the risk of Type 2 diabetes is lower in younger offspring of first-generation migrants of South Asian and African-Caribbean groups, but they still retain higher rates than white groups of European ancestry (Farmaki et al, 2020).

Type 2 diabetes is also more prevalent among children and adolescents from BME groups than children of white European ancestry (Ehtisham et al, 2001; Haines et al, 2007). Figures show that the incidence of Type 2 diabetes among Asian children is nearly seven times greater (and nearly four times greater for black African and African-Caribbean children) than that of white children in England and Wales (Candler et al, 2018). Furthermore, the incidence of this condition is continuing to rise among ethnic minority children, with South Asian children being the worst affected over the last decade (Candler et al, 2018).

When we look at health-related risk factors for cardiovascular disease broadly, there are still higher rates among BME groups. For example, levels of obesity and physical inactivity are higher among those categorised as black, Asian and other groups. Notably, data from the Active People survey from 2017–18 shows that people from these ethnic groups were more likely than average to be physically inactive, at 31%, 29% and 30% respectively; in contrast, people from the white British, white other and mixed ethnic groups were less likely than average to be physically inactive, at 24%, 23% and 18% respectively (Public Health England, 2020). There are differences across ages among ethnic groups, with lower levels of physical inactivity among younger generations compared to that of older generations. However, among people in the 35 to 44 age group, in every ethnic minority group except Mixed, they are more likely than average to be physically inactive (Public Health England, 2020).

Research about the prevalence of obesity among ethnic minority adults is disparate (El-Sayed et al, 2011). However, more studies indicate that the prevalence of obesity among ethnic minority adults in the UK is generally higher than other groups. Black adults, in particular, are identified as having a higher prevalence than white groups in the UK (Sutaria et al, 2019). For example, between 2017 and 2018, Black adults (76.3%) were the most likely out of all ethnic groups to be overweight or obese (Public Health England, 2020). Gender differences in obesity have been identified within ethnic minority groups. Notably, for men in London, the odds of obesity are higher among black ethnic groups compared with white British/Irish males and lower among Chinese, Indian, Bangladeshi and white men. Among women in the same region, all ethnic groups except Chinese and white Other had increased odds of obesity compared with white British/Irish women (Sutaria et al, 2019).

Research also shows that there are higher rates of obesity among children from most ethnic minority groups between the ages of 10 and 11 years (Public Health England, 2020). However, children from certain ethnic minority groups are more commonly identified as having the highest prevalence. Notably, South Asian children in the UK have been found to have higher levels of obesity than white British children (NHS Digital, 2017; Shah et al, 2020), with Pakistani and Bangladeshi children aged 11 years experiencing the highest obesity levels (26% and 28% in Pakistani and Bangladeshi respectively) within this group (NHS Digital, 2018). African and African-Caribbean children are also commonly identified as having higher rates of obesity prevalence, with recent National Child Measurement figures showing the highest rates among these children in both reception and year 6 (NHS Digital, 2020). These findings are relatively similar to those reported prior to 2011.

It is important to note that standard Body Mass Index (BMI) classification figures, commonly used for measuring obesity, Type 2 diabetes and heart disease, are not appropriate for understanding risk in black and Asian ethnic minority groups. Figures presented that illustrate differences in these conditions and risk across ethnic groups are at a lower BMI than the white population, with lower BMI intervention thresholds advised by the (then) National Institute for Health and Clinical Excellence (NICE, 2013) for Black and Asian groups.

Mental health

There are persistent ethnic health inequalities in mental health conditions among BME people in the UK that do not appear to have changed significantly since 2011. Numerous studies and reports still show that people from these groups are at a much greater risk than white British people (National Inclusion Health Board (NIHB), 2014; O'Mahony, 2017; NHS Digital, 2018b; PHE, 2018; Millan and Smith, 2019; Nazroo et al, 2019; Race Disparity Unit, 2019b; Race Equality Foundation, 2019). Notably, BME groups are more commonly diagnosed with a severe – psychosis-related – mental illness, such as schizophrenia, and this is particularly the case for black African-Caribbean or black African people (Nazroo et al, 2019; Edge et al, 2020).

Certain BME groups also have more adverse pathways to mental healthcare, as they are more likely to be compulsorily detained under the Mental Health Act and they are less likely to receive alternative therapies (Mental Health Task Force, 2016). An Independent Review of the Mental Health Act, commissioned by Theresa May in 2018, found disparities in the way that BME patients were treated within the mental healthcare system, with data indicating that they were disproportionately subject to restraint on wards. This disparity has been identified as being mostly significant for black African and black African-Caribbean groups (Edge et al, 2020), notably men (Race

Disparity Unit, 2019b; Keating, 2019). This is evidenced in the Cabinet Office *Ethnicity, Facts and Figures* data (Race Disparity Unit, 2019b), showing that black or black British people (black African-Caribbean and black African) were over four times more likely to be detained under the Mental Health Act than white people. For example, figures also show that black Caribbean people had the highest rate of detention under the Mental Health Act out of all ethnic groups. This is 3.7 times as high as the rate for White British people (Race Disparity Unit, 2019b). They are also less likely to access alternative therapies to manage their mental health (Glover and Evison, 2009). Black men are the most detained ethnic group, but they are less likely to receive psychological interventions and are, therefore, at greater risk of readmission (Watkins et al, 2010; De Maynard, 2014).

While this data implies that BME women experience lower levels of mental health conditions than ethnic minority men, research shows that they still experience higher rates than white British women (Race Disparity Unit, 2017); this varies across ethnic groups, with Black women being identified as having higher rates of common mental health disorders than other groups (Asian, Mixed and other women). However, it has been argued that common mental disorders are still highly prevalent among South Asian women, but diagnosed less frequently (Anand and Cochrane, 2005; Husain et al, 2006; Karasz et al, 2007; Mukadam et al, 2011; Wittkowski et al, 2011).

More recently, improved research evidence on the mental health status of adult Gypsies, Roma and Travellers has found that they have higher levels of stress, anxiety and depression than white non-Traveller groups (National Inclusion Health Board, 2014; O'Mahony, 2017; Public Health England, 2018; Millan and Smith, 2019; Race Equality Foundation, 2019). This is coupled with significantly higher rates of suicide among these groups, notably men (Abdalla et al, 2010). The accumulation of stress and anxiety from issues specifically affecting Gypsies, Roma and Travellers – such as living in non-permanent accommodation; stigma and discrimination; economic pressures; high unemployment among men; the changing role of men as providers for the family; and their relationship with the police – have been identified as key reasons for these rates (McGorrian et al, 2013; Thompson, 2013; O'Mahony, 2017; O'Donnell and Richardson, 2018).

These figures on mental health detentions and pathways for BME groups should always be considered with caution. The reasons behind the recording of mental health and detention outcomes are often more complex; involving longstanding experience of discrimination and structural factors that include deprivation, racism, racialisation and racial stereotyping (Keating and Roberston, 2004; Karlsen et al, 2005; Cooper et al, 2008; Wallace et al, 2016). Researchers have suggested that social injustice and racism may explain why the diagnosis of mental health and the detention figures are higher among certain BME groups. For example, although black Caribbean people are more likely to be treated for psychosis, they may not be any more likely to have such an illness (Keating, 2007). Racial stereotyping and misunderstanding of cultural expressions of anxiety or distress among psychiatrists and clinicians can lead to increased detentions for these groups. This is particularly the case for black men, who can become demonised as 'Big, Black, Bad and Dangerous' in mental healthcare and criminal justice settings, and thus experience fewer opportunities for different diagnoses or therapies (Walker, 2020: 44).

COVID-19

More recently, the COVID-19 pandemic has highlighted the persistence of ethnic health inequalities among groups from different minority ethnic backgrounds. These include not only a higher risk of contracting the condition, but also a higher risk of death.

COVID-19 results from Public Health England compared to UK Biobank data, have shown that the risk of testing positive for COVID-19 is higher among BME groups in the UK (Niedzwiedz et al, 2020). Specifically, Black and South Asian groups have been identified as being more likely to test positive for COVID-19, and those of Pakistani ethnicity were at the highest risk among South Asian groups. Black groups were also most likely to have COVID-19 diagnosed, with the lowest diagnosis rates being in white ethnic groups (Public Health England, 2020; Lacobucci, 2020a). Recent figures compiled by the UK's Intensive Care National Audit and Research Centre (ICNARC, 2020) also suggest that of nearly 5,000 people critically ill with COVID-19 in England, Wales and Northern Ireland whose ethnicity was known, 34% were from BAME backgrounds. This is concerning, given that people from these ethnic minority groups only make up 14% of the population of England and Wales (Office for National Statistics, 2011).

The risk of death from COVID-19 among BME groups is also significantly higher than other groups. The latest Public Health England (2020) report, *Covid-19: Review of differences in risks and outcomes*, illustrates this; notably that being black and from a minority ethnic background is a major risk factor. This disparity is evident even after accounting for the effects of age, deprivation, region and sex. People of Chinese, Indian, Pakistani, Other Asian, Caribbean and Other black ethnicity had between 10% and 50% higher risk of death when compared to White British people (Lacobucci, 2020a) The Public Health England (2020a) review also shows that people of Bangladeshi background face twice the risk of death compared with people of white British ethnicity. The Office for National Statistics (2020) figures for COVID-19 accounting for deaths beyond hospital settings, showed similar findings. The figures for the risk of death for people from black groups were nearly double (1.9 times higher), when compared with people from white groups.

The Public Health England (2020a) review also shows that co-morbidities are strongly linked to the increased risk of death from COVID-19, with higher rates of these conditions among BME groups being linked to higher rates of death. For example, people of Bangladeshi and Pakistani background have higher rates of cardiovascular disease than white British people. Notably, the review shows that among reported BME COVID-19 deaths there is a higher prevalence of 'diabetes, hypertensive diseases, chronic kidney disease, chronic obstructive pulmonary disease and dementia than all causes of death'.

Recent data for COVID-19 risks also shows differences in sex between ethnic groups. Men from ethnic minority groups are at a greater risk of contracting COVID-19, but also have a higher risk of death. Notably, the Office for National Statistics (2020) figures show that men of Bangladeshi or Pakistani background were 1.8 times more likely to die than white men, while BME women were 1.6 times more likely to die than white women.

However, these risks increase for pregnant BME women. Notably, a number of reports have also shown that more than half of pregnant women who were admitted to hospital with COVID-19 in the UK were black and from minority ethnic backgrounds. For example, research by Knight et al (2020b) shows that 56% of pregnant women from BME groups were admitted to UK hospitals with COVID-19 between March and April 2020, where 25% and 22% of women were Asian and Black respectively. This is deeply concerning, given that maternal health problems among BME women are already significantly higher than among other ethnic groups.

It is also important to draw attention to the impact that COVID-19 restrictions have placed on the mental health of BME groups. For example, there has been a significant increase in levels of depression, anxiety and loneliness experienced by BME women (Nuffield Foundation, 2020). For pregnant BME women, reduced access to support from maternity services has had the impact of social isolation and increased mental health concerns. The restrictions on access for partners, visitors and other supporters of pregnant women in maternity services imposed by the Conservative government during the summer of 2020, exacerbated the existing inequalities in access for pregnant BME women (Germain and Yong, 2020). It was not until December 2020 that women were able to attend prenatal appointments, scans and delivery suites with partners, visitors and other supporters (NHS England, 2020). However, this access was not facilitated for all women across the country. Despite changes made to NHS guidance in November 2020, NHS trusts were able to tailor their policies to their local situation, and therefore equal access to support at all times during their maternity journey was not facilitated until December 2020. The potential impact of these restrictions on BME women's mental health specifically, is yet to be evidenced in published studies, but it is likely that this has had a significant impact on their maternity journeys.

Drivers of disparities for risk of death of COVID-19

The impact of COVID-19 has duplicated existing health inequalities among ethnic minority groups and, in some cases, has increased them. The causes are yet to be fully understood in public health reports, but the Public Health England review (2020a), discussed earlier, proposes that they are a result of a 'combination of factors'. It has been suggested that BME groups are at an increased risk of contracting the virus because they are more likely to live in urban areas, in overcrowded households and in deprived areas. They are also located in jobs that expose them to a higher risk. They are also more likely to face 'poorer outcomes' after catching the virus, because some experience health conditions and co-morbidities that are more common among certain BME groups. However, at the time of writing, the review has been criticised for not clearly identifying any underlying reasons for the higher COVID-19 infection and mortality rate among BME groups.

Furthermore, recommendations on how to address the disparities and evident ethnic inequalities were published sometime after this initial report. It has been found, that a key part of the review was removed prior to public dissemination by the Conservative Party (Bhopal, 2020; The Guardian, 2020; Moore, 2020). A section was missing that appeared in a draft version circulated a week prior to publication with responses from more than a thousand organisations and individuals, many of them suggesting that the wider determinants of health, such as discrimination and poorer life chances, played a part in the greater COVID-19 risk for ethnic minority groups (Bhopal, 2020; Moore, 2020). Office for National Statistics (2020) COVID-19 figures, published at that time, take into account factors including age, geography, socio-demographic characteristics (such as deprivation), health and disability. Despite adjusting for these factors, the risk of death related to COVID-19 is still significantly higher among BME groups.

The missing section of the Public Health England report has since been published (16 June) as *Beyond the Data: Understanding the impact of COVID-19 on BAME groups* (2020b), and looks specifically at the social and structural determinants of health that impact on disparities in COVID-19 incidence and mortality in BME groups. Alongside a rapid literature review, it provides a summary of stakeholder insights into the factors believed to be influencing the impact of COVID-19 on BME communities and strategies for addressing these. The review outcomes suggest that the wider determinants of health have an impact on COVID-19 outcomes for BME groups. Specifically, the review states that overcrowded housing, financial vulnerability, reliance on public transport, racial discrimination, occupational risk, unequal access to healthcare, and residency in high population centres, are central to explaining why some ethnic groups experience greater risk incidence and mortality from COVID-19.

Despite these findings, more research is required to fully understand the correlation between COVID-19 ethnicity and wider determinants of health. What is also not discussed at depth in this review – and is often not explored in other research about ethnic health inequality – is an intersectional approach that examines how the wider determinants of health may occur simultaneously and thus are impactful on unequal health outcomes for BME groups.

The importance of taking an intersectional approach is discussed further in Chapter 3, but for now let's examine some of the wider determinants of health that have been identified in health research and reports, to ensure that we understand and examine them in our future practice.

Why are ethnic health inequalities occurring in the UK?

There are a number of factors that influence health outcomes, but these are largely outweighed by the overwhelming impact of social, cultural and economic factors, for example the material, social, political and cultural conditions that shape our lives and our behaviours (Marmot and Allen, 2014).

The Marmot Review (Marmot, 2010) and the Marmot Review 10 Years On (Health Foundation, 2020) demonstrate these factors as the most important influences on health and health inequalities. These include social, cultural, political, environmental and economic factors, and are commonly referred to as the 'wider social determinants of health'. The health and social care system is also included (Marmot, 2010). Marmot (2010) identifies six key areas as wider social determinants: the quality of experiences in the early years; education and building personal and community resilience; good quality employment and working conditions; income; healthy environments; and priority public health conditions.

While the Marmot Review (2010) draws attention to health inequalities and the social determinants, critics have argued that ethnicity and race issues are rarely discussed and are not recognised as being prominent (Chouhan and Nazroo, 2020). It is only now, in the recent COVID-19 Marmot Review, that this has been considered (Marmot et al, 2020).

In light of this paucity, researchers have argued that wide-ranging health inequalities for ethnic minority groups can be attributed to the likelihood of them being disadvantaged across all aspects of society. For example, people within an ethnic minority group are more likely to experience poverty, have poorer educational outcomes, be unemployed, and be discriminated against. These, in turn, are understood as the wider social determinants for poor ethnic health outcomes, and can be embedded in structural racism (to be discussed later in the chapter).

The development of the Equality Act 2010, mentioned earlier, has played an important part in giving legal recognition to ethnic health inequalities and the impact of the wider determinants of health. It became a legal duty for the Secretary of State for Health, for NHS England and for Clinical Commissioning Groups to reduce health inequalities and to comply with the Equality Act 2010. With race being included as a protected characteristic within the Act, public sector bodies within health now have a duty to address ethnic health inequalities to improve equality in healthcare and practice for all.

This Act has led to increased guidance for public health practitioners on recognising the wider determinants of health for ethnic minority groups. For example, the Public Health England (2018) report *Health inequalities*, discussed earlier, is one of the first national resources to examine ethnic health inequalities and its causes. This report illustrates the wider social determinants of health that occur for ethnic minority groups, and includes evidence on areas such as employment, housing, income, discrimination and social networks. However, it does not provide evidence on directly associated relationships between health status and these wider determinants. Having said that, it does encourage those in public health to recognise these wider determinants, when trying to understand why ethnic health inequalities occur and how they can be confounded.

Socioeconomic status

Socioeconomic position or status is understood as a wider determinant of ethnic health, because it can lead to increased exposures to health risk factors that in turn cause disease. Socioeconomic factors including deprivation have been recognised more recently as one of the wider determinants of health that impact on the increased risk of COVID-19 for certain BME groups (Public Health England, 2020b). This association of socioeconomic status factors, such as income, with a health risk factor or disease is also likely to be confounded by other socioeconomic variables, such as educational attainment. Before examining how socioeconomic status impacts on other ethnic health outcomes, it is important to look at the complexity in using this concept to understand ethnic health inequalities.

Within health research, the concept of socioeconomic status – and the factors included that impact on health – varies extensively (Stronks and Kunst, 2009). In UK health research, it is most frequently referred to as the social and economic conditions within people's lives. Common indicators of socioeconomic status include deprivation, education, employment status or quality, and income. Research examining health inequalities often includes an examination and inclusion of a deprivation index (Berthoud and Bryan, 2011), such as the Index of Multiple Deprivation. This measures deprivation in income, employment, living environment, health, education and training. It also considers barriers to housing and services, and crime within an area. Others have used an alternative index, such as Townsend's index of area deprivation, which is based on four factors: unemployment; car and home ownership; household overcrowding; and material deprivation (Townsend, 2017). Although there are common indicators of socioeconomic status, the World Health Organization (WHO, 2004: 5) recognises that 'there is no right answer' as to what should be included as a socioeconomic factor, and that a variety of measures of socioeconomic position or status could be included to examine ethnic health inequalities. What is important to recognise is that the concept is not without its limitations, and that there are considerable differences in the measures included when examining ethnic health inequalities.

Research has shown that the socioeconomic status of ethnic minority groups is associated to poor health. One of the starkest examples is infant mortality and socioeconomic position. For example, Kroll et al (2020: F56) have found that socioeconomic circumstances contribute to ethnic variation in infant mortality among preterm babies. Among 32–36 week births, all ethnic minority groups had a higher risk of death from congenital anomalies than white British women. Additionally, risks of death from congenital anomalies and combined rarer causes increased with deprivation.

Research has also shown that low socioeconomic status of ethnic minority groups is associated to other poor health outcomes. For example, Raisi-Estabragh et al (2020) have found a significant association between greater material deprivation, BME ethnicity, male sex and higher odds of COVID-19. If we look at cardiovascular health-related risk factors, Higgins et al (2019) have found a strong association between BME migration status and obesity (waist circumference) that is attenuated partly by socioeconomic status.

This association between low socioeconomic status of ethnic minority groups and poor health is not surprising in the UK, given that ethnic minority groups, in general, do have a lower socioeconomic status than the majority population (Nazroo, 2003). However, the association between socioeconomic status and poor health outcomes can vary by ethnic group (Allik et al, 2019) and gender (Knight et al, 2020a). For example, research by Allik et al (2019) found that socioeconomic inequalities in health are truly different across ethnic groups. Notably, in their research, Pakistani people living in Scotland were more likely to experience poor health in the least deprived areas, particularly at ages 45 and above. Furthermore, maternal mortality figures show that the rates of maternal death in pregnancy are higher among certain ethnic minority women, notably Asian and black women, and these rates remain high among those women living in more deprived areas and thus located in lower socioeconomic positions (Knight et al, 2020a).

Research has also found that there are inequalities between the level of income that ethnic minority groups and white British groups experience. This can impact on ethnic health inequalities. Ethnic minority groups on average also earn less than white British groups. Notably, Office for National Statistics (ONS, 2019) data shows that employees in the Black African, Caribbean or black British, Other and White Other ethnic groups on average earned 5% to 10% less than their White British counterparts between 2012 and 2018. In London, percentage difference in median hourly pay between people of a White ethnicity and all those who belong to an ethnic minority group is largest in London at 21.7% (ONS, 2019). Employees in the Pakistani and Bangladeshi ethnic groups experience greater inequalities in pay differences than any other group, earning the lowest median hourly pay. Bangladeshi ethnic groups are the worst hit, on average, as they earned 20.2% less than White British employees (ONS, 2019). Younger generations (16–30 years) from ethnic minority groups tend to have narrower pay gaps than older groups, but inequalities in pay still remain when compared to white British groups. These income disadvantages impact on health outcomes for ethnic minority groups, because there are fewer opportunities to look after their health, and thus the risk of disease increases (Nazroo, 2003).

Research has also shown that ethnic health inequalities are impacted by employment type (Joseph Rowntree Foundation, 2017). This is evident, for example, among NHS staff. While ethnic minority groups are employed widely within the NHS (40%), they are not equally distributed across roles (Moberly, 2018; Millner et al, 2020). Milner et al (2020) examined the 2017 NHS Digital workforce statistics on NHS Hospital and Community Health Service staff groups working in trusts and clinical commissioning groups in England, and found race-ethnic pay disparities. Specifically, they found that although Chinese people working in the NHS are more likely to be employed as doctors than other ethnic groups, they are less likely to be employed as consultants. Black ethnic minority groups working in the NHS were doubly disadvantaged, having a low prevalence among doctors and, within the doctor groups, as consultants. In contrast, white people employed by the NHS as doctors, were the most likely to be employed as consultants than any other ethnic group.

As discussed earlier, ethnic minority groups are disproportionately represented in high-risk keyworker roles that have been at an increased risk of COVID-19 and death. This is particularly apparent in large urban areas and for those in keyworker healthcare roles. For example, BME workers make up a disproportionately large share of keyworker sectors, such as transport and health and social care, in London and experienced the highest rates of COVID-19 diagnosis and mortality (Labour Force Survey, ONS, 2019; Public Health England, 2020a).

The analysis of income by ethnic groups is much more complex than has been discussed here, as there are many more dimensions of income to be considered (Platt, 2007). Furthermore, there are more complex differences in these measures according to ethnic group (Nazroo, 2003), gender and religion (Karlsen et al, 2020). However, what is common in key pieces of research data, is that there is economic disadvantage among certain ethnic minority groups in the forms of income and occupational type. This can impact on opportunities to look after health, and thus can heighten the risk of poor health. This is not to suggest that poor health results from poor choices, but rather that poor health can be the result of economic or socioeconomic disadvantage (Health Foundation, 2020). An adequate income can help people to avoid stress, and to access experiences and material resources that provide opportunities needed for a healthy life, which affect long-term physical and mental health. Those in lower-paid professions and high-risk roles have fewer opportunities to protect their health, and this drives inequalities in health outcomes for ethnic minority groups.

Structural racism and discrimination

The social and economic disadvantages experienced by ethnic minority groups such as those discussed earlier, are embedded in structural forms of racism – or what is more commonly defined as 'structural racism' (Gee and Ford, 2011). Ethnic health inequalities are perceived by some sociologists, Critical Race Theorists and health researchers as a form of, or a by-product of, structural racism (Bonilla-Silva, 1996; Ford and Airhihenbuwa, 2010; Gee and Ford, 2011). For example, it has been argued recently by Marmot (2020) that the disproportionately high number of black British people currently being killed by COVID-19 compared to those from white groups in the UK, is due to structural racism. So, what does structural racism mean and how can it help health researchers and health practitioners?

Structural racism refers to the processes and ways in which societies foster racial discrimination through systems in society such as housing, education, employment, income, healthcare and criminal justice (Bailey et al, 2017). These patterns and practices in turn reinforce discriminatory beliefs, values and distribution of resources, and perpetuate racial group inequity. Structural racism differs from other forms of racism – such as institutional racism, which refers to micro-practices within and across institutions that recurrently put a racial group at a disadvantage. In contrast, structural racism refers to the system-level, macro-processes across an entire society. The ideologies, practices, processes and institutions that function at this macro-societal level construct and reinforce unequal access to power and to life opportunities along racial lines. Structural racism is therefore embedded in societal-level institutions, policies and practices, and influences ethnic health inequalities through multiple pathways (Gee and Ford, 2011). For example, some argue that the social and economic disadvantages faced by Black ethnic minority groups are a contributory source to their higher risk of psychotic illness (Qassem et al, 2015). Their experiences of racialised Black identities therefore increase risk of economic adversity, unemployment, discrimination and harassment – and thus contribute to poor mental health outcomes.

While structural racism is recognised and acknowledged in health research, policy and practice as being influential to ethnic health inequalities, more research focuses on discrimination or racial prejudice in interpersonal interactions as the primary driver of these inequalities. Notably, research has linked discrimination to a broad range of conditions, including heart disease, mental health and obesity, as well as to low birthweight, COVID-19 and premature mortality (Gee et al, 2009; Williams and Mohammed, 2009; Gee et al, 2012; Priest et al, 2013; Public Health England, 2020b). Williams et al (2019), in particular, have shown the direct effects of racial discrimination on physical health. In the context of mental health, Karlsen et al (2005) have shown that the risk of psychosis was doubled for those who reported an experience of racist verbal abuse or physical assault. More recently, it has been suggested in the COVID-19 Public Health England (2020b: 33) report that the high levels of mortality for BME NHS staff could be attributed to 'racism, bullying and harassment at work', because BME staff were 'reluctant to speak up about issues (such as PPE shortages), [and thus] placed them at higher risk'.

Researchers have also argued that ethnic minority groups are more likely to suffer discrimination that occurs in their negative experiences in healthcare services and this impacts on poor health (Nazroo et al, 2009). For example, ethnic minority groups are more likely to experience primary care GP services negatively. The NHS (DOF) (2019a) shows that 'patients least likely to report a positive experience were from the Bangladeshi (72.6%), Pakistani (72.8%) and White Gypsy or Irish Traveller (72.9%) groups'. These experiences of GP services do not seem to have improved. For example, NHS DOF (2019a) also shows that BME patients are least likely to report a positive experience of GP services over a six-year period. Notably, 'Bangladeshi (73.7%), Pakistani (72.3%), Indian (76.0%) and Chinese (75.8%) ethnic groups – were consistently among the least satisfied groups over a 6-year period since 2011/12'. Patients also express dissatisfaction with their experiences in hospital settings. The NHS DOF (2019b) shows that patients from Bangladeshi, black African-Caribbean and other black backgrounds were the least satisfied with hospital services in 2017–18. Bangladeshi groups were the least satisfied of any ethnic group in 2017–18 and they were the least satisfied in each of the two years covered (2016/17–2017/18). These experiences regularly include racial stereotyping and discrimination.

Studies of maternity care in hospital settings have also reported that women from minority ethnic groups report poorer experiences of care than white British women (Henderson et al, 2013; Jomeen and Redshaw, 2013). In particular, South Asian women and black women have reported experiences of maternity care that entail stereotypical and discriminatory behaviour (Firdous et al, 2020). As discussed earlier, current research in the UK also shows that in maternity, mortality is highest among Black women; they are five more times likely to die in pregnancy than white women (Knight et al, 2018). Furthermore, Black and Asian pregnant women have recently been identified as being at a higher risk of COVID-19 and more likely to die than any other ethnic group (Knight et al, 2020b).

These health inequalities appear partly attributable to the failure to provide equitable care to ethnic minority groups in the UK. This can be in services not offered, in services badly given, or in services provided that are culturally inappropriate for the client group. The disparity in receipt of services has been identified as a factor contributing to adverse maternal and neonatal outcomes (Lewis, 2007).

Conclusion

It is evident that ethnic health inequalities have existed for some time in the UK. In this chapter, a brief examination of research evidence and public health reports has shown that these inequalities exist in health outcomes for cardiovascular disease, Type 2 diabetes, COVID-19, mental health and health-related risk factors such as physical inactivity and obesity.

Although there have been few national surveys examining specifically the health outcomes of BME groups since 2003, current data indicates that people from certain BME groups continue to be worst affected by poor health and these conditions. The recent global COVID-19 pandemic has raised awareness of the existence of ethnic health inequalities, and has arguably led to closer attention by public health agencies, government and researchers for the need to record more accurate health outcome data by ethnic group. Importantly, it has also highlighted the diverse drivers and wider determinants of health that exist and impact on the health and healthcare access for BME groups. That being said, it is highly evident that there is still a paucity of national public health resources that examine ethnic health and its causes.

3

Improving research on race, ethnicity and health inequalities

In the previous chapter, a number of differences in healthcare outcomes by ethnicity were examined and attention was drawn to some of the existing ethnic health inequalities in the UK and why they occur. However, it has been widely acknowledged in both health research and applied healthcare practice that ethnic health data is hampered by poor quality data. Thus, it is argued in this chapter that improvements need to be made to improve the visibility of ethnic minority groups in research and public health reports and in the methods utilised to research them (Bhopal, 1997, 2007). It is argued that by improving the equality and cultural competency practices of health researchers, we can improve visibility of diverse BME groups in health research data and practice.

As discussed in Chapter 1, there are common issues that occur in the recording of ethnic health data due to misunderstanding of the meaning of ethnicity and/or race (Williams, 1994; Møllersen and Holte, 2009), there are variations and inaccuracies in the recording of ethnicity (Aspinall, 2003, 2011, Comstock et al, 2004; Saunders et al, 2013) and there is a failure to record ethnicity (Public Health England, 2020a, 2020b, 2020c). This is actually complicated further by limited understanding of appropriate equality and cultural competency practices that are required to improve visibility of ethnic minority groups in research and health monitoring (Benoit et al, 2005; Mateos et al, 2009). But what are the implication of this for understanding of ethnic health inequalities and the drivers – and what more can we do to address these issues?

Problems with existing data: misunderstanding the meaning of ethnicity and race and the distinction between these concepts

As discussed in Chapter 1, the concepts of ethnicity and race are contentious terms that are often misunderstood and used interchangeably in health research and applied practice (Craig et al,

2012). The more common general conceptions recognise that ethnicity refers to one's cultural and social identity and difference, and race is a biological referent that refers to one's skin colour (Malik, 1996; Mason, 2000; Mulholland and Dyson, 2001; Johnson et al, 2019).

Despite these general conceptions, race classifications are combined with ethnic identity in health research and practice to label various ethnic minority groups (Bhopal and Donaldson, 1998; Comstock and Castillo, 2004; Bhopal, 2007, 2013). As discussed earlier, these are informed by the categories utilised by the ONS and national Census that encapsulate what is commonly perceived as the multidimensional nature of ethnicity (nationality, country of birth, language, religion, national or geographical origin and skin colour). This conception of ethnicity and ethnic groups/classifications is utilised in health practice, such as NHS monitoring records and the Health Survey, as diagnosis for disease, treatment of disease and to measure patterns in health service access (Bhopal, 2007, 2013). They are also embedded in some health intervention guidelines (for example NICE, 2011).

While a commonly understood term for ethnicity is needed for diagnosis and recording, we must recognise that problems arise in utilising the multidimensional concept of ethnicity. It can lead to misconceptions that race and ethnicity are interchangeable, and that the determinant of ethnic health disparities is due to race and biology – and not to any ethnic differences driven by social, cultural and economic factors. This can potentially lead to more studies of ethnic health being driven by a genetic or biological deterministic model that assumes that race is a valid biological category. For example, this implies that the health of ethnic minority groups is determined primarily by racial biological factors (Cooper and David, 1986; Krieger, 1987).

Researchers have also found that the terms used for ethnicity and race are infrequently defined in health service research, and race is recurrently employed in a routine and uncritical manner to represent ill-defined social and cultural factors (Williams, 1994; Bhopal and Rankin, 1999; Møllersen and Holte, 2009; Bhopal, 2013). For example, Møllersen and Holte (2009) investigated how the concept of ethnicity and its variable was used in mental health research – in theory, in measurement and in classification criteria – between 1990 and 2004. They found that the ethnic variable was incompletely reported across studies. There was also evidence of confusion regarding which individual or social characteristics ethnicity refers to, and researchers were often vague about what measures they used to measure ethnicity. This is not particularly helpful, when policy makers, commissioners and researchers try to look for explanations for differences in health outcomes between ethnic minority and white groups.

As discussed earlier, the current Conservative government and Public Health England team have recently been criticised for failing to publicise a report in which the impact of the structural and social factors on higher rates of COVID-19 and mortality among ethnic minority groups had been acknowledged (The Guardian, 2020; Moore, 2020), thus implying that these outcomes are driven by genetic and/ or biological deterministic factors.

Failings, variations and inaccuracies in the recording of ethnicity and ethnic groups

One of the most common problems that impacts on our understanding of ethnic health inequalities, is the invisibility of ethnic minority groups in research due to the incompleteness of ethnicity recording. Ethnicity is often not captured in public health reports, NHS monitoring data, or research data (such as clinical trials and survey data). For example, current COVID-19 data collected via Hospital Episode Statistics, clinical vaccine trials, and NHS COVID-19 trackers have failed to record ethnicity.

At the start of the pandemic, testing sites recorded demographic information of patients, such as age and location, but did not record race and/or ethnicity. Also, the Public Health England (2020a) *Covid-19: Review of differences in risks and outcomes* did not have information on the ethnicity of 3,555 of the 102,466 patient deaths recorded. Similarly, the Public Health England (2020c) *Rapid Investigation Team (RIT) preliminary investigation into COVID-exceedances in Leicester* contains significantly incomplete or 'unknown' information on ethnicity, despite utilisation of this data to impose the first city lockdown in July 2020. This can be explained partly by the lack of recording of ethnicity at testing sites in Leicester and via the online registration process.

The incompleteness of ethnicity recording ultimately impacts upon the quality and depth of research that has been – and can be – carried out. But, most importantly, it also impacts upon the ability to understand ethnic health inequalities, such as COVID-19 and its latest COVID-20 mutation, and respond to the needs of ethnic minority groups (Public Health England, 2020b). Campaigns have more recently taken place to improve the underrepresentation of ethnic minority groups in COVID-19 studies and vaccine trials; however, while they are disproportionately affected by the virus, they are still underrepresented. For example, research by the National Institute of Health Research

(NIHR) shows that 622,978 people have taken part in COVID-19 studies across the UK, but only 9.26% of ethnic minority groups have been involved. Furthermore, only 5.72% (1,509 participants) have taken part in vaccine studies (NIHR, 2020).

The implications of this are potentially significant, as it can discourage BME people from participating in the vaccination of the COVID-19 virus. For example, research indicates that individuals who identify as BME groups are more reluctant than white British groups to take the current COVID-19 vaccines (Fisher et al, 2020), despite being the ethnic group more likely to die from the virus. Bell et al (2020) also found that Black, Asian, Chinese, Mixed or Other ethnic groups were almost three times more likely to reject a COVID-19 vaccine for themselves and their children than White British, White Irish and White Other participants.

Some studies are investigating this further and have found that reluctance is due to feelings of uncertainty about the differential effects of the vaccine on ethnic minority groups. There is uncertainty about the speed of its development and overall distrust of healthcare provision, given that so few BME groups have taken part in the vaccine trials (Gramlich and Funk, 2020). While studies of this nature are telling, much further research is needed to understand more about these concerns from the perspectives of BME groups in the UK.

This is important, because current media reporting has focused heavily on the unwillingness of BME groups to take the vaccine and less on the structural racism and discrimination that may have fuelled these concerns. Over-reporting of this reluctance to receive the vaccination can contribute to further stigmatization, in which BME groups are perceived as problematic and once again hard to reach.

However, BME groups interviewed for this book wanted more information and transparency on vaccine trials from the Department of Health, before they made decisions about whether to take the vaccine. In light of this, researchers could work more with BME groups to improve their underrepresentation in clinical trials and research. However, this should not focus solely on encouraging BME groups to come forward to take the vaccine via community champions and role models who have had the vaccine (Hanif et al, 2020), but rather should do more to provide inclusive clinical trials, in which a larger number of BME people are included in the research.

One of the additional problems that impacts on the invisibility of ethnic minority groups in research is the diversity in recording ethnicity (Møllersen and Holte, 2008). As discussed in Chapter 1, there are significant variations and inaccuracies in the defining and categorising of ethnic groups in health research and health practices. This can occur in a number of ways.

First, broad classifications of ethnic groups are used and often do not reflect the heterogeneity within each ethnic group. Notably, ethnic groups can be classed in an entire BME/BAME category that is compared to white British groups. Similarly, black, Asian or South Asian ethnic categories are used without further detail on the different ethnic groups within these (Aspinall, 2003, 2011). For example, some research studies commonly categorise African and African-Caribbean and, in the US, African American into a black ethnic group. However, this does not account for the various countries of origin or descent within the black African or Caribbean group, despite the variations in culture, practice and behaviour between these smaller groups (Comstock et al, 2004). As a consequence, results from many different studies cannot be compared on equal terms, to understand ethnic health inequalities (Bhopal, 2007; Mateos et al, 2009).

Second, smaller, less visible ethnic minority groups, such as the Gypsy, Roma and Travellers, new migrants and asylum seekers, are missed by current ethnicity recording. As discussed in Chapter 1, Gypsy, Roma and Travellers groups are now officially categorised and legally recognised in official Census and health data recording as an ethnic minority group, yet separate classifications for this group are often missing (Public Health England, 2020c). They are still commonly categorised into a white ethnic group category in health monitoring and research (Cabinet Office, 2019b). Furthermore, when a separate category for Gypsies and Travellers is given, they are often subsumed into one ethnic group category, despite differences of language, history and culture (Condon et al, 2019). Groups within this, such as Irish Travellers, can then be placed within a homogeneous group that may include Roma Travellers who experience different beliefs, histories, cultures and health practices (Cabinet Office, 2019b).

Third, the methods utilised for recording of ethnicity are often inaccurate. While self-reported ethnicity methods are advised in healthcare and research as the gold standard of ethnic monitoring (Aspinall, 2011), healthcare practitioners and researchers will not commonly record the ethnicity of a patient or participant, and this can cause inaccuracies in NHS records. Saunders et al (2013) found that healthcare practitioners incorrectly record ethnicity in NHS routine ethnicity data, because it differed to that self-reported by patients in patient surveys. These inaccuracies can arise because there is often a lack of understanding among healthcare practitioners and researchers of how to record a person's ethnicity (Mateos et al, 2009). Furthermore, there is uncertainty about which people belong within a specified group (Benoit et al, 2005) and a general lack of cultural competency in how to ask for this information.

Research, equality practices and cultural competency

It has been widely acknowledged that there is a lack of understanding in both healthcare and research on how to collect equality monitoring data and how to be culturally competent in monitoring ethnicity and/ or race (Jones and Kai, 2007; Mateos et al, 2009). Measures to address this in NHS healthcare have increased significantly due to the Equality Act 2010, which requires public and private services to demonstrate equal treatment across all areas of employment and delivery of care, including access to care provision. Furthermore, incentives to improve ethnicity coding under the Quality and Outcomes Framework in primary care, have helped to improve monitoring.

However, in health research there is less emphasis on addressing this. Furthermore, there are few UK-based studies that look at the equality monitoring practice and cultural competency of researchers involved in health research. As discussed in Chapter 1, there are numerous studies that report on what researchers can do to engage hard-to-reach BME groups (Liljas et al, 2017; Condon et al, 2019; Liljas et al, 2019; Prinjha et al, 2020), but there is a paucity of research that specifically examines the equality practices of health researchers.

In response to this gap and to requests from ethnic minorities who have been involved at the Centre for BME Health, University of Leicester, I have been leading National Institute of Health Research (NIHR) ARC East Midlands research with a team of researchers that examines health researchers' practice regarding the equality of participant involvement in the planning, delivery and implementation stages of applied health research. The aim is to review their involvement in new equality monitoring practices, equality impact assessments and measures taken to address the inclusion of underrepresented and seldom heard ethnic minority groups in research. PPI data indicate an unwillingness of researchers from white ethnic groups to engage in equality monitoring processes and a lack of understanding of its relevance or significance to their proposed research. Furthermore, there is significantly limited knowledge of central terms, including 'race' and 'ethnicity', and there are misconceptions about BME groups.

The remaining findings are yet to be reported due to delays for the COVID-19 outbreak and lockdown. However, there are still some existing studies in the US and some in the UK that report on existing cultural competency education and training for health researchers to improve the invisibility of minority groups in research (Papadopoulos and Lees, 2002; Lawless et al, 2014). Specifically, Lawless et al (2014) implemented and evaluated a cultural competency training programme for clinical and health researchers in Ohio, in the US. They too recognised the paucity of cultural competency programmes for researchers and research on evaluating their implementation. They found that a cultural competency educational programme (Conceptual Framework and Model: Experiential Learning Framework and The Cultural Competence and Confidence Model (Jefferys, 2006)), with a neighbourhood visit approach, improved the cultural knowledge, attitudes and behaviour of health researchers. There were significant changes in both the way researchers think about the community and the way the researchers conduct research. Furthermore, the involvement and inclusion of community members from ethnic minority backgrounds in the planning phase was vital to improving the understanding of people from diverse ethnic, racial backgrounds. Specifically, community representatives from numerous neighbourhood institutions were able to design and plan the activities that the researchers would be involved in.

What needs to be recognised here, is that improvements to the recording and monitoring of data should to be coupled with research and practice that improve the equality and cultural competency practices of health researchers. This can help to improve the visibility of diverse ethnic minority groups in health research data. Furthermore, the more we know about ethnic minority groups, the more that can be done in policy and by clinical commissioners to improve health, services provision and inequalities in access to them. Research completed should not be tokenistic, in which a few ethnic minority individuals are consulted or only included in small parts of the research process. Furthermore, it should be completed *with them*, with consideration of their input, perceptions and experiences – as opposed to being *on them*.

Conclusion

It has been evidenced in both this chapter and the previous chapter that ethnic health inequalities exist and are disproportionately experienced by ethnic minority groups. The COVID-19 pandemic has brought further attention to the presence of health differences in healthcare outcomes by ethnicity and race.

However, further measures need to be taken to improve the visibility of ethnic minority groups and BME groups in healthcare research and practice. It can no longer be assumed that these groups are hard to reach and less visible, but rather that data recording of health by race and ethnicity and the methods utilised to research ethnic minority groups are inequitable. There are still significant problems in the recording and monitoring of ethnicity and its classifications. This contributes to an invisibility of ethnic minority groups in health research and public health data. There is also limited recognition of the diverse and intersecting explanations of observed differences in health outcomes according to ethnic group. This is unfulfilled in health and ethnicity research, and needs to be urgently improved.

What also needs to be addressed is the infancy of equality monitoring and training on the importance of collecting equality data and how to achieve this in UK health research. This has also led to inaccuracies and inconsistencies in what we know about health outcomes by ethnic group and the drivers for these conditions.

What we can do is complete more research and improve healthcare practice that examines the equality monitoring practices and cultural competency of researchers and healthcare staff involved in health research and services. We can also improve the training that informs these practices. However, this can no longer take the form of online cultural competency and equality, diversity and inclusion training that is taken too infrequently, lacks input from ethnic minority groups and is often forgotten or misunderstood.

4

The importance of intersectionality

This chapter focuses on current academic definitions of 'intersectionality' and highlights why the term is important for the delivery of health interventions for ethnic minority groups. In recognition of recent research on intersectionality, additional dimensions of difference and marginality for ethnic minority groups are discussed here (Reimer-Kirkham and Sharma, 2011; Mwangi and Constance-Huggins, 2017; Collins and Bilge, 2020).

A brief exploration of some of the current health interventions and studies that employ an intersectional approach is provided. However, it is argued that few in the UK facilitate a focus on this approach. Furthermore, few apply the theory to examine the interconnected ways in which multiple aspects of identity impact on health and access to healthcare interventions for ethnic minority people (Tomalin et al, 2019).

This chapter sets the context for Chapter 5, in which a research case study is presented about why intersectionality theory is important for addressing misconceptions about ethnic minority people as being hard to reach in health intervention delivery.

Intersectionality theory

'Intersectionality' refers to the intersections and interconnectedness of social identity, and recognises that inequalities cannot be explained by one identity, condition or location (Crenshaw, 1989, 1991). While the concept and theory were originally intended to address the effects of sex/gender and race/ethnicity within the legal profession, it has been extended to other domains, notably in the study of health (Bowleg, 2012).

However, as yet, it has not been widely employed in the study of health inequalities (Smith et al, 2016). Despite this, use of this approach is needed and important, because it can allow health researchers and practitioners to focus on the ways in which features of social identity are interrelated and can be detrimental to health and healthcare access (Heard et al, 2019). It also allows for the 'study of health at different intersections of identity, social position processes of oppression or privilege, and policies or institutional practices' (Bauer, 2014: 10). This approach is also vital for understanding ethnic health inequalities because, as outlined in Chapter 2, the various axes of inequalities are often studied in isolation (Bowleg, 2012). Furthermore, the 'lived experiences of [health] that involves ongoing intersections across all of these different axes are often misunderstood' (Smith et al, 2016: 6). So now let's look at the concept of intersectionality and current approaches that can assist us in the study of ethnicity and health.

The concept of intersectionality was originally coined by the legal academic Kimberlé Crenshaw and arose in the late 1980s from Critical Race Studies (Crenshaw, 1989; Cho et al, 2013). The concept allowed for recognition of the intersections of race and gender for black women – notably Black African American women – and demonstrated the multiple systems of stratification and its simultaneous impact (Cole, 2009). It was an approach that drew attention to the intricacies of difference and the commonalities of sameness in the context of anti-discrimination (Carbado et al, 2013). Specifically, Crenshaw (1989, 1991) exposed how a singular approach to women's oppression challenged legal thought, knowledge development and social justice movements (Giritli Nygren and Olofsson, 2014). The concept has since developed and been interpreted in many ways by different disciplines, practitioners and policy makers. However, the most common approach defines intersectionality: 'as the power relations of race, class, and gender … [that] are not discrete and mutually exclusive entities, but rather build on each other and work together; and … these intersecting power relations affect all aspects of the social world' (Collins and Bilge, 2020: 2).

There are also differences in the analytical frameworks employed. More commonly, they utilise a heuristic and explanatory framework that investigates social injustice and seeks to solve social problems (Bowleg, 2012; Collins and Bilge, 2020). Notably, Collins and Bilge (2020: 2) argue that, 'as an analytic tool, intersectionality views categories of race, class, gender, sexuality, class, nation, ability, ethnicity and age – among others – as interrelated and mutually shaping one another. Intersectionality [therefore] is a way of understanding and explaining complexity in the world, in people and in human experiences'.

Intersectionality offers a theoretical and analytical framework for health researchers, practitioners and commissioners (Bauer, 2014; Bowleg, 2012; Smith et al, 2016; Heard et al, 2019). Bowleg (2012), in particular, argues that the framework encompasses core tenets that are pertinent to the study of public health and applied healthcare practice. She argues that social identities are not autonomous, but are multiple and intersecting. Moreover, it can encourage further analysis of people who have been oppressed and marginalised historically and who are often seldom heard.

In light of Bowleg's recommendation, we can see how intersectionality offers opportunities to look more closely at the relationship between social identity and health for ethnic minority groups. Smith et al (2016: 102), in particular, argue that it allows health researchers and practitioners to examine the 'multifaceted aspects of identity' and its position in society that impacts health outcomes and behaviour. This encourages movement beyond assumptions that certain ethnic minority groups are homogeneous and that the drivers for health inequalities are similar across groups. It also offers an opportunity to look at 'the axes of power' that impact on the wider determinants of health and inherent disadvantages experienced by these groups (Smith et al, 2016).

Importantly, Smith et al (2016) argue that the latter shifts attention from commonly held biological deterministic approaches to health that attributes health and health behaviour to individual factors among minority groups. This is somewhat similar to Bowleg's argument for the application of intersectionality to public health. Bowleg (2012: 1268), too, argues that 'multiple social identities at the micro level (i.e., intersections of race, gender and SES) intersect with macrolevel structural factors (i.e., poverty, racism and sexism) to illustrate or produce disparate health outcomes'. By adopting this approach, we can therefore, not simply assume that ethnic health inequalities are attributable to individual or biological factors, but rather to intersecting dimensions of difference.

New approaches to intersectionality in the study of health now include additional dimensions of difference and marginality to recognise the multifaceted aspects of identity for ethnic minority people (Reimer-Kirkham and Sharma, 2011; Mwangi and Constance-Huggins, 2017). Instead of utilising unitary approaches, in which one principal category of social position is of primary research interest, multiple single categories are examined (Bauer, 2014). These include, for example, geographical location and religion. Specifically, Mwangi and Constance-Huggins (2017) argue that to advance Black women's health, an intersectionality approach should be integrated into health research and practice, and should go beyond the usual intersection of race and gender to include geographical rurality. They suggest that in the US, rural settings in non-urban areas can impact health outcomes. They argue that black women living in these areas can experience greater levels of poverty, limited access to healthcare and racial segregation, when compared to women living in urban areas.

Reimer-Kirkham and Sharma (2011) also recommend that religion is added to gender, race and class to understand how ethnic minorities experience inequalities in access to healthcare. They argue that religion for some ethnic minorities involves processes of racialisation, oppression and marginalisation that are experienced as part of their gender, race and class. This is discussed further in Chapter 5.

By looking at these additional dimensions, we can take the approach of Smith et al (2016) and move beyond categorising ethnic groups as homogeneous. For example, people within one ethnic minority group can have differentiated experiences of religious affiliation and geographical residence that may impact on health outcomes.

Preventative health and lifestyle interventions

There are various preventative health and lifestyle interventions that focus on improving the health of ethnic minority groups in the UK. However, as yet, there are still few in the UK that facilitate an applied focus on the application of intersectionality theory and the interconnected ways in which intersections of social identity impact on health and access to services for ethnic minority people (Heard et al, 2019; Tomalin et al, 2019). Lack of this approach in intervention delivery can, in part, explain why ethnic minority groups are commonly perceived as being hard to reach in healthcare and intervention services.

If we recognise 'the axes of power' that influence the health and disadvantages experienced by ethnic minority groups, we can also identify the barriers and wider determinants of health that impact their access to health interventions (Smith et al, 2013). Therefore, instead of assuming that being hard to reach is the fault of ethnic minority groups, it encourages analysis of the structural, social, economic and political factors and axes of power that impact on involvement and engagement in interventions. It thus requires greater attention on those in more advantageous or privileged positions who yield the axes of power (Smith et al, 2013; Heard et al, 2019) and who commission and deliver these interventions.

Numerous researchers outside the UK have argued for this approach to be applied to health and lifestyle interventions for minority populations (Griffith et al, 2011; Bowleg et al, 2013; Huang et al, 2020; Heard et al, 2019). Notably, Griffith et al (2011) provide recommendations on how intersectionality should be incorporated in the delivery of obesity and physical activity interventions for black African American men. They argue that there are multiple social determinants of health that intersect with gender and masculinity for these men. These include: 'poverty, poor educational opportunities, underemployment and unemployment, incarceration, and social and racial discrimination [and] all of these factors challenge and influence the capacity of poor men and men of colour to achieve and maintain good health' (Griffith et al, 2011: 421). Therefore, these factors should be considered in future interventions.

Similarly, Bowleg et al (2013) have argued that an intersectional approach can be employed to HIV prevention interventions for black African American men. They argue that there has been a dearth of health prevention interventions that recognise the intersections of identity that black African men experience and the impact these have on their health risk. However, most of the research and intervention have focused on women and not considered the additional dimension of sexuality for black men. They argue that few HIV prevention interventions address 'the social-structural issues that these men perceive to be most relevant to their lives' and apply this to intervention delivery and evaluation (Bowleg et al, 2013: 10). Through qualitative interviews with black African American men, they found that an intersectional approach is important for understanding these men's 'multiple intersecting social identities (e.g., race, gender, socioeconomic status and sexual orientation) and reveal interlocking systems of ... oppression (e.g., racism, sexism, classism, heterosexism)' (Bowleg et al, 2013: 8) that impact on their HIV risk and access to interventions. Specifically, they argue that these men's experiences of 'racial discrimination and racial microaggressions, unemployment, incarceration, and police harassment' (Bowleg et al, 2013: 7) should inform interventions and thus 'alleviate the intersectional burdens of "the uphill battle" of being a black man at the macro social-structural level' (Bowleg et al, 2013: 11).

Researchers have also argued that the approach should be applied to health promotion strategies and interventions designed for ethnic minority groups. Notably, Halkier and Jensen (2011) argue for a contextual theoretical perspective that includes multiple social conditions and dynamics − a combination of practice theory and intersectionality. They found that the promotion of healthier eating among Pakistani Danes needs to be delivered in recognition of the multiple intersections of social identity such as class, gender and ethnicity, and how they impact on how the ethnic minority group involved in their research practise healthy eating.

Researchers have also applied an intersectional approach to recruitment of participants and evaluation of the intervention delivery. For example, Heard et al (2019b) utilise an interactive drama and focus groups as a practical tool for applying intersectionality to analysis of an intervention of intimate relationships with young people in Samoa – experiencing high rates of partner violence and alienation from sexual and relationship health promotion. An intersectionality approach was used to inform the data collection and thematic analysis of the participants' identity and its interaction with social and cultural systems. For these young people, 'age, gender, religion and sexuality interact with social hierarchies and power structures, socially prescribed gender norms, family structures and globalisation' (Heard et al, 2019b: 1) and ultimately their health and engagement with health promotion. Heard et al (2019b) therefore argue that the intersectional approach is important for the development of prevention strategies to address the root causes of intimate partner violence experienced by young people in Samoa.

Other researchers have examined how intersectionality has been applied to the recruitment of minority participants to mental health interventions and which methods are most successful. For example, Huang et al (2020) have completed a systematic review that examines the extent to which intersectionality theory has been integrated into the recruitment of sexual minority populations to mental health interventions in Hong Kong. They also examined which type of instrumental methods are more commonly used to ensure intersectionality in evaluation of the intervention. They found that community-based participatory research was used more commonly and successfully.

Despite recommendations for the use of intersectionality theory in delivery and evaluation of health interventions in various countries (Bowleg, 2012; Bowleg et al, 2013; Lui et al, 2016), this approach is still in its infancy in the UK. The few studies that exist in the UK have argued for the application of intersectionality theory to understand ethnic health inequalities. They often focus on how the theory can be used to examine the multifaceted aspects of identity, and how they impact on health outcomes and access to healthcare services or interventions for ethnic minority people.

For example, Semlyen et al (2018) interviewed Muslim gay men living in London to understand their experience of health service use and how intersectionality impacted on inequalities in access for these men. In their findings, they found that an additional dimension of marginality in intersectionality (religion) was relevant. For these men, the complex intersection of religious, ethnic, gender and sexual identities impacted on their identity disclosure dynamics with healthcare practitioners, and led to negative consequences of assumptions made by practitioners, be these heteronormative or faith-related. The authors draw attention to implications of this research for healthcare practitioner training and interventions to connect intersectionality with health inequalities. Specifically, they argue, 'healthcare professionals need improved understanding of intersecting identities and how to be able to be non-judgemental and to empathise with and understand them'. This study suggests that further training in understanding of intersectionality is needed for those delivering health services and interventions. This research also illustrates that without recognition of the intersectionality approach, these minority groups will continue to be perceived as hard to reach and non-engaging in health services and interventions.

Despite this study, there are still very few UK studies that look at how the approach can be applied in the evaluation of health promotion or prevention interventions designed for ethnic minority groups. This brings us to the case study in the next chapter, in which an intersectional approach is applied to evaluation of a culturally tailored diabetes awareness and prevention programme for ethnic minority groups.

5

Case study: "We are not hard to reach, you are just not reaching us!" Understanding intersectionality and the prevention and management of Type 2 diabetes among British African-Caribbean women

This case study chapter presents the lived experiences of (n=30) British African-Caribbean women (18–75 years), who engaged with a culturally tailored and community-based diabetes risk awareness and prevention programme. The programme is appraised via focus groups with these women. By listening to the voices of these women, this case study chapter shows that health services have largely treated these British African-Caribbean women as 'hard to reach'. However, these women do not categorise themselves as 'hard to reach', but rather argue that health services "are not reaching" them, by assuming that health practices are equally applicable and effective for all women.

It is argued that the design and delivery of previous services fail to recognise how intersections of these women's identities impact on their health and access to services. Recommendations are given to improve the development of health interventions by involving British African-Caribbean women in the design and provision of culturally tailored interventions in their communities and by applying intersectionality theory and methodological frameworks.

Introduction and background

Type 2 diabetes

Type 2 diabetes mellitus (T2DM) is one of the most common chronic illnesses in the United Kingdom (UK) (Diabetes UK, 2010, 2018). Some 3.8 million people are estimated to have both types of diabetes, but approximately 90% of diabetes cases are T2DM (Diabetes UK,

2010, 2018; Public Health England, 2016). It is a long-term condition that causes the level of sugar (glucose) in the blood to become too high due to the body not making enough insulin, or the insulin it is making is not being used properly (Diabetes UK, 2018). In total, it is estimated that 10% of the National Health Service (NHS) budget is spent each year on treating diabetes and its complications (Hex et al, 2012).

The central causes for this condition are being overweight and inactive and/or having a family history of the disease (Diabetes UK, 2010, 2018). The risk of developing T2DM can be reduced by changes in lifestyle and health-related behaviours, such as diet and physical activity (Sargeant et al, 2018). Early diagnosis and careful management are vital, to prevent the condition and associated complications such as heart attack, stroke and kidney disease.

Risk and prevalence of Type 2 diabetes in BME groups

As discussed in Chapter 2, Black and Minority Ethnic (BME) groups in the UK have higher rates of T2DM and develop the condition up to 10 years earlier than White European populations (Chaturvedi, 2003; Diabetes UK, 2010; Khunti et al, 2013). British African-Caribbean populations are a higher risk of developing T2DM (Tillin et al, 2013) and experience associated higher rates of mortality and morbidity (Riste et al, 2001) than White Europeans. In the case of this research, British African-Caribbean refers to people who self-assign their race as Black or mixed, who have ancestral links to Africa via the Caribbean and are of Caribbean descent living in the UK (Agyemang et al, 2005; Higginbottom, 2006). However, in adopting this term, it is recognised here that there are significant variations in culture, traditions, beliefs and languages between and within the Caribbean islands and therefore do not intend to homogenise the participants.

The prevalence of T2DM is three times more common in people of African-Caribbean ethnic origin (Diabetes UK, 2012; Public Health England, 2014) than white British. Furthermore, it is estimated that approximately 40%–50% of all African-Caribbean people in the UK will develop the disease by age 80, compared with only one in five of European descent (Tillin et al, 2013). The condition affects about 5.7% of the African-Caribbean population, compared with around 4.4% of the general population (British Heart Foundation, 2001; Forouhi et al, 2006). There is also a higher prevalence and incidence of risk factors among this group, including hypertension and obesity (Health Survey for England, 2004). Additionally, morbidity from diabetes-related complications for African-Caribbean people is highest in those with low socioeconomic status (Bennett et al, 2015).

African-Caribbean women and Type 2 diabetes

African-Caribbean and South Asian men in the UK have the highest rates of T2DM incidence when compared to White European men (Ferguson et al, 2018). However, African-Caribbean women, have a greater risk of developing T2DM than White European women (Sproston and Mindell, 2004), because they carry greater levels of fat around the trunk or middle and have an increased resistance to the effects of insulin (Tillin et al, 2013).

Lifestyle risk factors for developing T2DM, such as obesity and inactivity, are higher in British African-Caribbean women than White European women (Pomerleau et al, 1999; Rowe and Chapman, 2000; Health Survey for England, 2004; Shoneye et al, 2011; Diabetes UK, 2016). While higher risk and prevalence rates for these women are more common over the age of 55 years (Health Survey for England, 2004), research indicates that diabetes risk factors (Saxena et al, 2004; Shaw et al, 2007) and prevalence are also high among African-Caribbean young women and girls (Candler et al, 2018).

The risk of developing multi-morbidities for BME women with diabetes is more common than for White European women (Mathur et al, 2011; Salisbury et al, 2011; Barnett et al, 2012). However, African-Caribbean women with T2DM are twice as likely as White European women to develop other long-term conditions like hypertension (Office of Population, Censuses and Surveys, 1996; Becker et al, 2006; Health Survey for England, 2004, 2017).

Hard to reach

As discussed in Chapter 2, the term 'hard to reach' is regularly adopted in health service provision to classify those populations who do not engage with clinical practice, primary care and prevention activities. They are also often conceptualised in this way in health research literature due to their invisibility in screening data (Douglas, 2018). There are research studies examining the experiences of marginalisation that BME women face in their access to health service provision (Arthur and Rowe, 2012). However, there are few studies that examine the experiences of British African-Caribbean women participating in diabetes prevention or lifestyle behaviour change programmes.

The invisibility of British African-Caribbean women in UK-based health research may be due, in part, to the inconsistent and inaccurate NHS record data relating to the ethnic origin of African-Caribbean women. While ethnicity monitoring is required in all healthcare provisions by NHS England, ethnicity and race are recorded inaccurately, as discussed in Chapter 3. It has been suggested that this is due to uncertainty and unease among healthcare staff as to how best to collect this data (Iqbal et al, 2012). Therefore, disparities that these women experience in healthcare access become difficult to monitor in the UK, because of the need for better ethnic monitoring data across the NHS and associated services (Szczepura, 2005). This can add to the organisational and structural factors that contribute to these women being perceived by health service providers as being 'hard to reach' in health interventions.

The term 'hard to reach' plays a debilitating role in 'othering' BME women within health interventions and health services, as it is often synonymised with other terms such as 'vulnerable', 'problematic', 'marginalised', 'hidden', 'forgotten', 'less worthy' and 'disadvantaged' (Flanagan and Hancock, 2010; Shaghaghi et al, 2011; Sydor, 2013; Ellard-Gray, 2015). It also often refers to those who may experience the highest risks of chronic disease, co-morbidities and mortality, and morbidity from ill health, yet are underserved due to lack of access to health services for social, economic and cultural reasons (Shaghaghi et al, 2011).

Categorising these women in this way is problematic, as it positions them as difficult and different to other White European women, but also reinforces their subordination and marginalisation in healthcare access (Bowleg, 2012). This and the inherent process of othering can potentially impact on the health of these women, as it can create barriers to access. For example, Bhopal (2012) argues that women perceived in this way, who feel unwelcome and have had negative experiences, are less likely to re-enter the health services system or associated provisions. For African-Caribbean women, perceptions of mistrust and racism escalate, as they come to believe that they are not given the same quality of service that White European women receive (Scott, 2001; Brown et al, 2007). Similar experiences have been evidenced in research with other minority women (Johnson et al, 2004).

Type 2 diabetes lifestyle behaviour change interventions for African-Caribbean women

Evidence suggests that lifestyle behaviour change interventions are suitable for driving diabetes prevention and improving management (Miners et al, 2012; Lewis et al, 2014). However, research shows that health outcomes for BME participants could be improved dramatically by culturally tailoring the programmes to the needs, health beliefs and concerns of BME participants (Brathwaite and Lemonde, 2017). Notably, studies have shown that there is a need for health, cultural and religious beliefs of African-Caribbean populations to be understood and incorporated into structured education programmes, to effect behaviour change (Scott, 2001; Noakes, 2010; Maynard et al, 2018). Additional behaviour change activities include exercise and dietary information that resonates with cultural habits (Moore et al, 2017). Furthermore, programmes delivered by role models within the community, and of the same ethnic origin, can increase opportunity and motivation to adopt recommended health behaviours (Moore et al, 2017). For example, Noakes (2010) found that African-Caribbean TD2M patients wanted African-Caribbean people treated with insulin, to help motivate and support them.

Existing lifestyle behaviour change interventions for BME women in the UK could also be improved, by recognising the socioeconomic factors that can potentially impact on managing personal health (Morris and O'Brien, 2011). For example, consideration can be given to differentiated work patterns and experiences. For example, African-Caribbean women are more likely to be in full-time work ('63% of African-Caribbean women compared to 54% of White British women'), yet they are also more likely to be working longer hours and facing discrimination in the workplace (Breach and Yaojun, 2017). Problems are also apparent for some of these women outside of paid work, with unemployment figures being high at 10%, which is double that of White British women at 5% (Breach and Yaojun, 2017). Additionally, many of these women are often located in less secure and in unskilled roles (Douglas, 2018) that provide limited opportunities for time to engage with health and lifestyle interventions.

With the exception of Moore et al (2017), few UK-based interventions have sought to recognise these differentiated experiences and to implement programmes that facilitate a focus on the multidimensional and interconnected ways in which gender, race, ethnicity and socioeconomic status impact on British African-Caribbean women's health. Most often, race, ethnicity and gender are treated as separated dimensions of social stratification and not recognised simultaneously in prevention interventions (Bowleg, 2012). However, it is recognised that culturally tailored interventions that are underpinned by appropriate theory, such as intersectionality theory, are an effective means of beginning to address the intersecting inequalities experienced by BME women to improve access and engagement (Bowleg, 2012).

Intersectionality

Black feminists have historically drawn attention to multiple oppressions of Black African American women, but after Crenshaw (1989, 1991) introduced the term 'intersectionality' in 1989, it was championed and widely adopted by other Black feminists (Collins, 1990; Nash, 2008). Black feminists welcomed this approach, as it allowed them to critique their marginality within feminism, arguing that the experiences being documented were largely about white women's experiences and not those of black African American women. They also sought to challenge the notion of a universal gendered experience, and argued that Black African American women's experiences were shaped by the interrelating and contradictory subtleties of race, gender, class, geography, and other axes of power and inequalities that work together in producing injustice (Collins, 1990, 2005; Collins and Bilge, 2016).

More recently, intersectionality has been drawn on to understand the health of black women in the US and Brazil (Bowleg, 2012; Caiola et al, 2014; Mwangi and Constance-Huggins, 2017; Hogan et al, 2018). It has also been utilised in research to evidence the health inequalities in hypertension and diabetes among minority women internationally (Gagné and Veenstra, 2017). However, as yet, few have applied this approach in order to understand the experiences of British African-Caribbean women participating in a T2DM lifestyle behaviour change programming, despite recognition of its need and potential applicability in health research (Bowleg, 2012; Edge, 2013; Douglas, 2016).

Despite this, there are central components of the intersectionality framework (Collins and Bilge, 2016) that are relevant for understanding the delivery of lifestyle behaviour change programmes for diabetes prevention and management and the inequalities that British African-Caribbean women face in accessing them. These include three core tenets identified by Bowleg (2012), but also the more recent work that extends intersectionality dimensions to other cultures and structures of difference, such as religion or faith (Reimer-Kirkham and Sharma, 2011) and rurality (Mwangi and Constance-Huggins, 2017). As discussed in Chapter 4, Bowleg (2012) argues that one of the core tenets involves recognition of multiple social identities that intersect with each other (Bowleg, 2012). This is important for understanding British African-Caribbean women, as they possess multiple disadvantages and several axes of oppression, all of which impact on their health, health risks and access to healthcare. Their socioeconomic positioning differs significantly to that of White European women, due to their differentiated positions in the labour market, longer working hours, discrimination and caring responsibilities (Breach and Yaojun, 2017) – all of which impact on their access and availability to attend diabetes prevention programmes.

In the early intersectionality work, Crenshaw (1989, 1991) focused on gender, race and class as indicators of marginality, but made recommendations for other cultures of difference and structure to be included (Nash, 2008; Collins and Bilge, 2016). This potentially includes other dimensions such as religion and/or faith that have been less considered in research. Here it is argued that religion and/ or faith can be important for understanding British African-Caribbean women's access to diabetes management and prevention services. Historically, religion and faith for British African-Caribbean women play a significant role in guiding their daily lives, but are also important for understanding their health beliefs and behaviours – and their impact on the inequalities in access to diabetes care (Brown et al, 2007). As discussed in Chapter 4, Reimer-Kirkham and Sharma (2011) argue that religion cannot be considered as a separate category of difference, but is integrated into people's everyday lived experience and thus impacts on oppression experienced. Religion can therefore be used as an additional factor that marginalises British African-Caribbean women and contributes to the othering processes that positions them as hard to reach (Reimer-Kirkham and Sharma, 2011).

Geographical location is also an additional dimension of oppression that can potentially impact on health outcomes and access to lifestyle behaviour change healthcare programmes for British African-Caribbean women. Evidence shows that African-Caribbean (98.2%) people are more likely than White Europeans to live in urban cities (ONS, 2018). Furthermore, British African-Caribbean women living in urban locations with low socioeconomic status have a higher risk and prevalence of T2DM (Diabetes UK, 2010).

Research also suggests that BME groups are represented in very small numbers in rural areas and are thus socially isolated. They lack social and community support found in other BME communities who are located in urban areas (Ray and Reed, 2005; Khan, 2012; Public Health England, 2017). The lower numbers of ethnic minorities in rural areas make them highly visible within rural communities, but can also make them invisible to service providers. Health promotion services that are catered specifically for them are limited, and incidents of rural racism can be more common (Khan, 2012).

In recognition of this recent research on intersectionality, religion/ faith and rurality are considered as additional dimensions of difference and marginality for British African-Caribbean women here in this research.

Methods

A case study design was adopted to understand the women's perceptions of the lifestyle behaviour change intervention (Yin, 2003). This design allows for in-depth examination of the women's experiences of the programme and its activities within its real-life context (Yin, 2009). Furthermore, it allows for questions about how the programme is being received on the ground and 'provides additional insights into what gaps exist in its delivery', all of which are aligned to the RE-AIM framework (Crowe et al, 2011: 4).

The case study approach is underpinned by constructivist positioning that 'focuses as much as possible on the participants' view' and recognises the importance of the subjective creation of meaning and the social construction of reality (Creswell and Poth, 2017: 24). It allows participants to tell their stories and describe their views of reality, thus enabling the researcher to better understand the participants' actions and experiences (Lincoln and Guba, 1985).

The principal research methods employed in this study were qualitative, semi-structured focus groups interviews. Qualitative methods were chosen, because they allow for the voices of participants to be heard and they are identified as an effective technique for co-designing a culturally tailored diet and lifestyle intervention for managing T2DM in African-Caribbean patients (Moore et al, 2017). The in-depth responses that can be obtained from qualitative questioning allows these women to communicate their identities (Edwards and Holland, 2013) and the intersections that impact on diabetes risk and prevalence, and their access to lifestyle behaviour change programmes.

Programme description

This programme was a 12-month behavioural lifestyle change intervention that sought to raise awareness and prevention of T2DM in BME groups. It was delivered by the Centre for BME Health at the University of Leicester, in partnership with the National Centre for Sports and Exercise Medicine at Loughborough University and the Leicester Diabetes Centre.

The intervention sought to improve physical activity levels, reduce sedentary behaviour and encourage healthy eating. These aims were informed by previous research delivered by the Leicester Diabetes Centre and Centre for BME Health, in which BME people within a UK city identified priorities around healthy lifestyle choices as being central activities for addressing their risk and prevention of T2DM. Open space qualitative focus groups were utilised in this previous research to access the understandings and needs of the BME communities. As the priorities were led and developed by the BME populations within these settings, the programme was delivered as a community-led model. The model is rooted in intersectionality theory, which recognises that communities should have a role in shaping decisions and circumstances that affect their wellbeing (Caiola et al, 2014). It also allows for recognition that health is socially and economically determined, and programme delivery should be informed by those who experience the intersections of marginality.

The programme builds on the previous research exploring the experiences, knowledge and understanding of T2DM and its prevention in minority ethnic communities. The intervention was targeted towards two of the seven BME groups who had participated in the previous study mentioned earlier. In this previous research, the majority of the participants had asked for the delivery of health promotion messages and community events to be targeted at specific ethnic groups. Furthermore, the community priorities for the intervention were to adapt and develop resources, to ensure that they were culturally sensitive to the differentiated BME populations. For example, this included developing and adapting culturally tailored guides for improving physical activity levels and reducing sedentary behaviour for each minority group.

Furthermore, the intervention sought to provide nutritional guidance. This included adaptation and development of the Eatwell Healthy Eating Plate (updated to *The Eatwell Guide* in 2016) (Public Health England, 2018) that is culturally relevant for their cultural food choices. *The Eatwell Guide* is based on nutrition advice, and is designed in a pictorial form (a plate) containing foods and drinks to help the communication of a healthy balanced diet to the population (Public Health England, 2018). For the programme, this included healthy eating booklets that included foods consumed specifically by British African-Caribbean people and South Asians.

The programme of activities included two large community health events, with activities for physical activity, nutrition (demonstrations) and sedentary behaviour that were delivered at the baseline and at the completion of the intervention. The first focused on the British African-Caribbean population and the second on the South Asian communities. A six-month development and implementation phase was led by a multi-ethnic Centre of BME Health staff that included researchers, diabetes dieticians, and community support workers – all of whom have existing partnerships and networks with the local BME communities.

The activities included free physical activity classes in community centres, and healthy eating workshops for each of the targeted populations. Culturally appropriate education about physical activity, alternative healthier foods and cooking methods via demonstrations in communities were acceptable ways of delivering such information. These were designed and differentiated for the specific minority groups, and took place in locations that were frequently attended by each of the British African-Caribbean and Bangladeshi communities and recommended by them. This included women-only aerobics sessions and healthy eating workshops in a Bangladeshi community centre that were culturally relevant for this community. For the British African-Caribbean participants, fitness sessions and culturally relevant healthy eating workshops were provided in an African/African Caribbean community centre located within the city centre. During these healthy eating workshops, dietitians provided healthy eating activities, and the women were served food cooked by local African-Caribbean chefs, who had adapted traditional Caribbean dishes to include less salt, sugar and fat but who also used alternative cooking methods (for example baking as opposed to frying). These sessions were devised to be inclusive for families and all ages, so children were also invited to attend. Seated-yoga sessions and Soca workout activity sessions were delivered by female African-Caribbean instructors at the community events and during the six-month implementation phase for the women.

The final community-based health event was intended to be a celebration event, providing the opportunity to bring all of the minority populations together to share what worked and what next. The event was targeted at both of the BME communities in response to the qualitative feedback given during the programme. While each of the BME groups wanted further attention to be given to their cultural needs within the programme, they requested to be with other minority populations that catered for each BME group. The intervention itself was delivered to over 1,000 people from South Asian and 1,000 British African-Caribbean communities within the East Midlands. Further details of the programme activities can be found in Table 5.1. This chapter focuses on the involvement of the British African-Caribbean women and the activities that were delivered for them.

Table 5.1: Programme activities

Phase 1: October 2016	Phase 2: Six-month development and implementation lead Centre for BME Health staff and community members, November 2016 to February 2017	Phase 3: March 2017
Community-based health event – Live Healthier Stay Healthier	Community-based activities – for South Asian men/women (500 attendees) • Women-only activities – aerobics • Healthy eating workshops – children and families	Celebration Live Healthier Stay Healthier event – for both BME groups, with opportunity to share what worked and what next (1,200 attendees)
Community-based health event – Live Healthier Stay Healthier	Community-based activities – African-Caribbean men/women (500 atendees) • Physical activity sessions – fitness, e.g. Soca dance sessions, boxing and circuit training • Seated yoga – women • Healthy Eating workshops – African-Caribbean children and families	

The RE-AIM assessment tool

The research evaluation of the programme was adopted and guided by the basic components of the RE-AIM framework. The aim of using this approach was to understand the reach, effectiveness, adoption, implementation and maintenance (Glasgow et al, 1999) of the programme that sought to raise awareness and prevention of T2DM among BME people.

RE-AIM is an assessment tool or framework that allows for the evaluation of health interventions (see RE-AIM.org, 2018). It was developed in 1999 by Glasgow et al (1999) and has multiple criteria related to health behaviour change. It has been utilised extensively in health intervention or programme evaluations for understanding both the perceptions of the communities who accessed the intervention and those who assist in its delivery. It has been used to evaluate T2DM prevention and management interventions (Toobert et al, 2002; Wozniak et al, 2015) for different BME populations (Bopp et al, 2007; Two Feathers et al, 2005; Whittemore et al, 2004). There are limitations in the application of the RE-AIM programme, as some research studies will draw on just one of the dimensions of analysis, while others will use all five dimensions of the framework (Gaglio et al,

2013). However, it is an effective framework for the development, tailoring and evaluation of interventions.

To recruit participants for the evaluation, open invitations were offered to all participants attending at the programme activities. Recruitment was face-to-face, with the researchers already visiting the programme activities and BME community engagement workers located in the Centre for BME Health (at the University of Leicester). In other cases, the research team and the community engagement workers distributed the study information, and potential participants responded to them. Convenience sampling was used, because participants were attending the programme activities and were available to participate (Hesse-Biber and Leavy, 2010; Green and Thorogood, 2018). Snowball sampling was also used to attract additional participants. Twelve qualitative focus groups (that averaged 60 minutes in length) were completed during the final phase of the programme with participants from each of the BME communities between the ages of 18 and 75 years.

Six of these were completed with the South Asian participants that included both males and females (n=180) and six were completed with the British African-Caribbean participants (n=30), all of whom were women. The findings from the latter are presented here in this book. The interviewees within the focus groups were provided with participant information sheets and consented to participate via informed consent forms. The ethical application was submitted and approved by the University of Leicester Research Ethic Committee.

Experienced qualitative researchers conducted the focus group interviews, audio recorded them, transcribed them verbatim, and took detailed interview notes. The community engagement workers supported the facilitation of these and provided language translation where required. Focus group interviews were adopted, because they allow researchers access to the 'shared social meanings, norms and how these are enacted' by the BME women (Green and Thorogood, 2018: 87). They also offer advantages that the interview cannot provide, notably allowing participants to interact with one another and share the oppressions and inequalities they may experience, particularly those experienced by African-Caribbean women in their interactions with health promotion services and the healthcare system. For example, Mitchell (2018) has found that when African-Caribbean women are given opportunities to engage in group enquiry with other African-Caribbean women, they experience positive feelings of self-worth and empowerment about their diabetes. Furthermore, women come together and connect on discussions about the lack of seriousness of diabetes and the effect is togetherness and empowerment (Mitchell, 2018).

The qualitative focus group interview guides were developed from the RE-AIM framework and previous studies that have developed interview questions covered from the dimensions of reach, efficacy, adoption, implementation and maintenance (Schwingel et al, 2016). The interview guide was piloted with members of the Centre for BME Health (at the University of Leicester), which included members of the public (via PPI sessions), organised by the community engagement workers and research staff members. Please see Table 5.2 for further details.

The five central research questions

The central research questions that inform this guide included the following:

1) Did the study effectively **reach** the number or proportion of people within BME communities who were willing to participate in the intervention?
2) Did the intervention **impact** (positively) on raising awareness and prevention of T2DM among BME communities?
3) Did BME people successfully **adopt** and undertake the intervention?
4) To what degree was the intervention **implemented** as originally intended, which includes consistency of delivery, time and cost?
5) Can the programme be **maintained** and sustained at individual and community-led levels?

To assess *reach,* research evaluations focus on the proportion of eligible people who participate in the intervention that can be accessed by measuring those who participated in the programme (Glasgow et al, 1990). For qualitative research this can include asking interviewees to estimate the number of participants who attended (Bopp et al, 2007), or simply whether they felt it reached eligible people, members and/ or communities. In the case of this research, we adopted the latter, thus asking participants if they felt it reached them and other African-Caribbean people within their community/ies.

Efficacy or effectiveness involves measuring the programme effects on important outcomes such as behaviour, lifestyle and health (Schwingel et al, 2017). This can include levels of physical activity, and/or dietary changes, and reduced risk of ill health. In the case of this research, participants were asked to comment on their own changes regarding levels of physical activity, sitting time, dietary changes, and increased awareness of T2DM and its risk. Participants who had T2DM were

Table 5.2: RE-AIM framework interview guide with community participants, staff and stakeholders

Actors: staff, participants and stakeholders	Examples of questions to assess specific RE-AIM components				
	REACH	*EFFICACY/EFFECTIVENESS*	*ADOPTION*	*IMPLEMENTATION*	*MAINTENANCE*
Participants Perceptions/interpretations and overall experiences of the **community members** who accessed the intervention.	• Do you feel the programme effectively reached members of your community/ies?	• How effective do you think the programme is in raising your **awareness of Type 2 diabetes** in the short term? • How effective do you think the programme is in **preventing your risk** of T2DM in the short term? • Did you notice any changes in your **lifestyle** after participating in the programme? Can you tell me what changed and what do you think caused you to change? • What do you think about your **eating and drinking habits?** Have you noticed any changes as a result of your participation in the programme? Can you tell me what changed and what caused this change?	• Do you feel the representative groups (BAME/ BAME communities)/ your communities successfully undertook the intervention? • Assessed via attendance during the three phase: Events 1 – community events; 2 – workshops; 3 – celebration event.	• Was there a workshop you were most interested in? Which was it? Why were you more interested in it? • Did you attend any of the workshops? If not, why not? If yes, please tell us what you thought about it. • What did you think about the activities and or materials you received? How often did you attend and/or use the materials you received? • In your opinion is/was there anything missing in the programme? • Was there a topic/area you were most interested in learning about during the programme? Which topic was it? Why were you most interested in it?	• Would you participate in this programme again? What motivates you most about participating in this programme? • If we were to offer this programme again would you recommend it to others? Why? What motivates you the most to recommend it to others? What reasons make you not want to recommend the programme to others?

(continued)

Table 5.2: RE-AIM framework interview guide with community participants, staff and stakeholders (continued)

Actors: staff, participants and stakeholders	Examples of questions to assess specific RE-AIM components
	• What do you think about your physical activity habits, have you noticed any changes as a result of your participation in the programme? • Can you tell me what changed and what caused this change? • To what extent has the programme changed your lifestyle behaviours, regarding physical activity, sitting time and eating behaviour? • Would you do anything to revise the programme? • Do you have suggestions or recommendations to attract others within your community to this programme in the future?
Staff Perceptions/interpretations of the **staff members** who assisted to deliver the intervention.	• Do you feel the programme effectively reached the number or proportion of people within BME/BAME communities who were willing and able to participate in the intervention? • How effective do you think the programme is/was in raising awareness of T2DM in the short term for BME/BAME groups? • How effective do you think the programme is/was in preventing their risk of T2DM in the short term? • Did you think the programme can change their lifestyle behaviours (physical activity, sitting time and eating behaviour) after participating in the programme? • Tell me your role in the programme? What were your thoughts on your experience of the programme? • As the programme developed, did your opinions about the programme change? How? • What did you enjoy most about your experience in delivering the programme? • What was it like to deliver the programme to the BME/BAME communities? • What do you think was most successful? Can you identify something that worked particularly well? Why do you think it worked well? • What were the challenges that you encountered during the programme implementation? Why do you think these happened and how did you overcome these? • If we were to run this programme again would you like to continue serving in your current role? Why? • Do you feel this type of programme can be maintained and achieve longevity within the BAME/BME community?

(continued)

Table 5.2: RE-AIM framework interview guide with community participants, staff and stakeholders (continued)

Actors: staff, participants and stakeholders	Examples of questions to assess specific RE-AIM components				
Stakeholders/ community support groups/church leaders/members Perceptions/ interpretations of the *stakeholders* who assisted to deliver the intervention.	• Do you feel the programme effectively reached the number or proportion of people within BME/ BAME communities who were/would be willing and able to participate in the intervention?	• How effective do you think the programme is/was in raising awareness of T2DM in the short term for BME/BAME groups? • How effective do you think the programme is/was in preventing their risk of T2DM in the short term? • Did you think the programme can change their lifestyle behaviours (specifically their physical activity, sitting time and eating behaviour) after participating in the programme?	• Do you feel the representative groups (BME/BAME communities) successfully undertook the intervention?	• What was it like to deliver the workshops? • What role did your organisation play in the implementation of this programme? • What are your thoughts about the programme? • What was it like to implement this programme? • Have you heard any comments from people affiliated with your organisation regarding the programme? What comments have you heard and from whom? • Do you have any suggestions or recommendation on how to implement this programme more effectively?	• What factors do you think affect the implementation of a programme offered to BAME/ BME communities? • What makes your organisation want to continue supporting this programme? • What do you think was most successful about your partnership with this programme? • Do you have any suggestions or recommendations for the future of the programme or this partnership?

asked to comment on whether their management of their condition had changed. In accordance with the constructivist approach adopted, the aim was to 'focus as much as possible on the participants view' and concomitant meanings (Creswell and Poth, 2017: 24).

Adoption concerns the representativeness of settings and people who deliver the programme (Glasgow et al, 1990). In this research, we asked participants whether they and the representative groups (BME communities) successfully adopted and undertook the intervention.

Implementation focuses on how well the programme adhered to the programme's principles and aims in its implementation (Glasgow et al, 1999; Bopp et al, 2007). This involved asking participants whether intervention was implemented as originally intended, which includes consistency of delivery as intended, time and cost. To understand this, we reminded participants about the aims of the programme and asked questions such as: What did you think about the activities and/or materials you received? How often did you attend and/or use the materials you received? Would you do anything to revise the programme? See Table 5.2 for further details. In the piloting of these questions, we received recommendations to include probes for cultural relevance. Notably, we were advised by the community engagement workers within the Centre of BME Health team to ask participants whether the culturally tailored activities met their cultural needs, which we included.

To assess *maintenance*, organisational and individual approaches can be taken to understand whether the programme activities and behaviours become part of routine practice (Glasgow et al, 1999). In this research, we focused on the extent to which the programme could become integrated into the activities of those involved in its delivery if continued, and the extent to which individuals would continue with the programme activities. Given that this project was only funded for one year, we asked participants what would be required for future maintenance at organisational and individual levels, if funded.

The qualitative data analysis was guided by the RE-AIM framework (Green and Thorogood, 2018). The framework provided pre-defined areas we wished to explore; however, we also wanted to remain open to discovering the unexpected, so a thematic analysis was adopted to analyse the data within these initial codes (Creswell and Poth, 2017). The first stage, therefore, involved analysis of the data and utilised the five dimensions of the RE-AIM framework as codes to group the data. This then involved open coding to examine for commonalities and difference (Strauss and Corbin, 1998) and the emergence of themes.

Stage two involved application of an intersectionality framework (presented in Table 5.3) to the themes identified in the focus groups with these women. The intersectionality template devised, is informed by Bilge (2009), who developed an intersectional strategy of analysis to understand masculinity among Montreal youth. Dimensions of the intersectionality template are flexibly applied as a methodological tool to understand the African-Caribbean women's comments. Importantly, this approach allows for investigation of the RE-AIM components through an intersectional lens. In this stage, the dimensions of intersectionality were identified deductively from the qualitative transcripts and utilised to create the final themes.

A diagrammatic map illustrating the codes, developed themes and application of the intersectionality framework for one of the RE-AIM dimensions is presented in Figure 5.1. This approach was adopted because it allows researchers to work with intersectionality; interpreting the data within the context of multidimensional forms of structural inequality (Bilge, 2009).

The methodological rigour of the study was addressed through various measures. Notably, team-based coding was completed to enhance the dependability of the findings (Brink et al, 2006). Each member coded the data independently, beginning with the central codes that were identified from the five aspects of the RE-AIM framework. The coders compared and contrasted how the open codes developed and were applied, and then reviewed them to ensure consistency. From here the coders identified and applied emergent codes that matched the views and terminology used by women. Intercoder agreement on how to apply the codes to the relevant text and the intersectionality framework was established between the coders, to avoid misrepresenting the women's experiences (Tolley et al, 2016). The trustworthiness of the researchers' interpretations was completed by revisiting the women, in a follow-up workshop. Research participants reviewed, validated and verified the researcher team's interpretations and conclusions – member checking was completed to ensure that the data and thematic analysis had not be misconstrued (Tolley et al, 2016). In accordance with the ethics, the participants were also reminded here that their anonymity would be assured in forthcoming publications and that their comments may inform the design of future interventions.

It was recognised by the research team that interviews with marginalised groups can serve to perpetuate inequalities for the participants (Edwards and Holland, 2013; Hesse-Biber and Leavy, 2010). This is particularly apparent where there are 'differences between

Table 5.3: Intentionality analysis template combined with RE-AIM framework

RE-AIM → Intersectionality dimensions → → →	Reach	Effectiveness	Adoption	Implementation	Maintenance
Gender	How is the *reach* of the programme impacted by the **gender** of the participant? How is the *reach* of the programme impacted by **gender** and other dimensions of intersectionality?	How is the *effectiveness* of the programme impacted by the **gender** of the participant? How is the *effectiveness* of the programme impacted by the **gender** and other dimensions of intersectionality experienced by the participant?	How is the *adoption* of the programme impacted by the **gender** of the participant How is the *adoption* of the programme impacted by the **gender** and other dimensions of intersectionality experienced by the participant?	How is the *implementation* of the programme impacted by the **gender** of the participant? How is the *implementation* of the programme impacted by the **gender** and other dimensions of intersectionality experienced by the participant?	How is the *maintenance* of the programme impacted by the **gender** of the participant? How is the *maintenance* of the programme impacted by the **gender** and other dimensions of intersectionality experienced by the participant?

(continued)

Table 5.3: Intentionality analysis template combined with RE-AIM framework (continued)

RE-AIM →	Reach	Effectiveness	Adoption	Implementation	Maintenance
Race and ethnicity	How is the *reach* of the programme impacted by the **race and ethnicity** of the participant?	How is the *effectiveness* of the programme impacted by the **race and ethnicity** of the participant?	How is the *adoption* of the programme impacted by the **race and ethnicity** of the participant?	How is the *implementation* of the programme impacted by the **race and ethnicity** of the participant?	How is the *maintenance* of the programme impacted by the **race and ethnicity** of the participant?
	How is the *reach* of the programme impacted by **gender** and other dimensions of intersectionality	How is the *effectiveness* of the programme impacted by the **race and ethnicity and** other dimensions of intersectionality experienced by the participant?	How is the *adoption* of the programme impacted by the **race and ethnicity and** other dimensions of intersectionality experienced by the participant?	How is the *Implementation* of the programme impacted by the **race and ethnicity and** other dimensions of intersectionality experienced by the participant?	How is the *maintenance* of the programme impacted by the **race and ethnicity and** other dimensions of intersectionality experienced by the participant?

(continued)

Table 5.3: Intentionality analysis template combined with RE-AIM framework (continued)

RE-AIM → Economic/ socioeconomic position	Reach	Effectiveness	Adoption	Implementation	Maintenance
	How is the *reach* of the programme impacted by the **economic/ socioeconomic position** of the participant? How is the *reach* of the programme impacted by the **economic/socioeconomic position and other dimensions of intersectionality?**	How is the *effectiveness* of the programme impacted by the **economic/ socioeconomic position** of the participant? How is the *effectiveness* of the programme impacted by the **economic/ socioeconomic position and other dimensions of intersectionality** experienced by the participant?	How is the *adoption* of the programme impacted by the **economic/ socioeconomic position** of the participant? How is the *adoption* of the programme impacted by the **economic/ socioeconomic position and other dimensions of intersectionality** experienced by the participant?	How is the *implementation* of the programme impacted by the **economic/ socioeconomic position** of the participant? How is the *implementation* of the programme impacted by the **economic/ socioeconomic position and other dimensions of intersectionality** experienced by the participant?	How is the *maintenance* of the programme impacted by the **economic/ socioeconomic position** of the participant? How is the *maintenance* of the programme impacted by the **economic/ socioeconomic position and other dimensions of intersectionality** experienced by the participant?

(continued)

Table 5.3: Intentionality analysis template combined with RE-AIM framework (continued)

RE-AIM →	Reach	Effectiveness	Adoption	Implementation	Maintenance
Age	How is the *reach* of the programme impacted by the **age** of the participant? How is the *reach* of the programme impacted by the **age** and other dimensions of intersectionality experienced by the participant?	How is the *effectiveness* of the programme impacted by the **age** of the participant? How is the *effectiveness* of the programme impacted by the **age** and other dimensions of intersectionality experienced by the participant?	How is the *adoption* of the programme impacted by the **age** of the participant? How is the *adoption* of the programme impacted by the **age** and other dimensions of intersectionality experienced by the participant?	How is the *implementation* of the programme impacted by the **age** of the participant? How is the *implementation* of the programme impacted by the **age** and other dimensions of intersectionality experienced by the participant?	How is the *maintenance* of the programme impacted by the **age** of the participant? How is the *maintenance* of the programme impacted by the **age** and other dimensions of intersectionality experienced by the participant?
Disability	How is the *reach* of the programme impacted by the **disability** of the participant? How is the *reach* of the programme impacted by the **disability** and other dimensions of intersectionality experienced by the participant?	How is the *effectiveness* of the programme impacted by the **disability** of the participant? How is the *effectiveness* of the programme impacted by the **disability** and other dimensions of intersectionality experienced by the participant?	How is the *adoption* of the programme impacted by the **disability** of the participant? How is the *adoption* of the programme impacted by the **disability** and other dimensions of intersectionality experienced by the participant?	How is the *implementation* of the programme impacted by the **disability** of the participant? How is the *implementation* of the programme impacted by the **disability** and other dimensions of intersectionality experienced by the participant?	How is the *maintenance* of the programme impacted by the **disability** of the participant? How is the *maintenance* of the programme impacted by the **disability** and other dimensions of intersectionality experienced by the participant?

(continued)

Table 5.3: Intentionality analysis template combined with RE-AIM framework (continued)

RE-AIM →	Reach	Effectiveness	Adoption	Implementation	Maintenance
Faith/religion	How is the *reach* of the programme impacted by the **faith/religion** of the participant? How is the *reach* of the programme impacted by the **faith/religion** and other dimensions of intersectionality experienced by the participant?	How is the *effectiveness* of the programme impacted by the **faith/religion** of the participant? How is the *effectiveness* of the programme impacted by the **faith/religion** and other dimensions of intersectionality experienced by the participant?	How is the *adoption* of the programme impacted by the **faith/religion** of the participant? How is the *adoption* of the programme impacted by the **Faith/Religion** and other dimensions of intersectionality experienced by the participant?	How is the *implementation* of the programme impacted by the **faith/religion** of the participant? How is the *implementation* of the programme impacted by the **faith/religion** and other dimensions of intersectionality experienced by the participant?	How is the *maintenance* of the programme impacted by the **faith/religion** of the participant? How is the *maintenance* of the programme impacted by the **faith/religion** and other dimensions of intersectionality experienced by the participant?
Rurality	How is the *reach* of the programme impacted by the **rurality** for the participant? How is the *reach* of the programme impacted by the **rurality** and other dimensions of intersectionality experienced by the participant?	How is the *effectiveness* of the programme impacted by the **rurality** of the participant? How is the *effectiveness* of the programme impacted by the **rurality** and other dimensions of intersectionality experienced by the participant?	How is the *adoption* of the programme impacted by the **rurality** of the participant How is the *adoption* of the programme impacted by the **rurality** and other dimensions of intersectionality experienced by the participant?	How is the *implementation* of the programme impacted by the **rurality** of the participant? How is the *implementation* of the programme impacted by the **rurality** and other dimensions of intersectionality experienced by the participant?	How is the *maintenance* of the programme impacted by the **rurality** of the participant? How is the *maintenance* of the programme impacted by the **rurality** and other dimensions of intersectionality experienced by the participant?

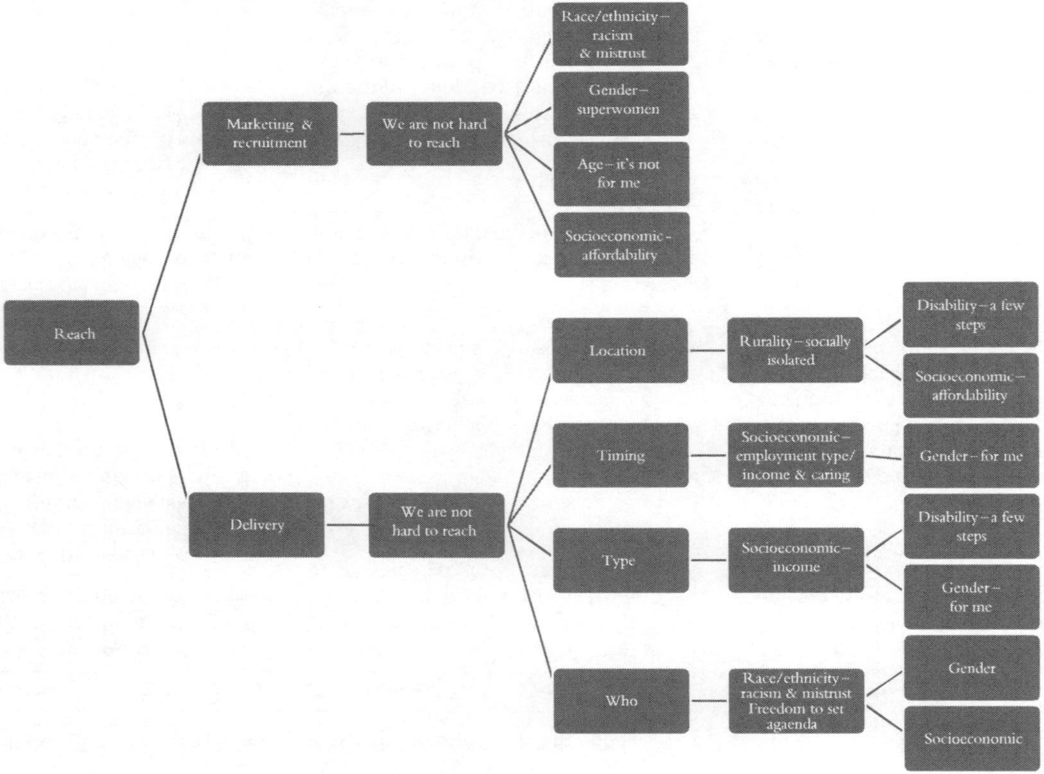

Figure 5.1: Diagrammatic map illustrating the codes and the developed themes with application of the intersectionality framework for one of the RE-AIM dimensions

the interviewer's "positionality" (social status, [race, ethnicity] and identity) in relation to an interviewee' (Edwards and Holland, 2013: 79). Through the process of reflexivity, it was acknowledged by myself (the central researcher) that I and interviewees both share membership of a marginalised BME group. As a mixed (Black/White) British-African female with African-Caribbean family members and children, it was important to recognise how my historical and cultural background could potentially shape my interpretation of these women's accounts. In accordance with the constructivist approach, I acknowledge how my own interpretations of the interview accounts flow from my personal experiences of marginalisation and invisibility in healthcare access (Creswell and Poth, 2017). However, the intention here was to acknowledge this, but also to make sense of the meanings that others (the British African-Caribbean Women) have of their interactions with the lifestyle behaviour programme and healthcare. To demonstrate this reflexive awareness in the research process, the interview interpretations and thematic analysis were open to outside inspection and verification from the study team via an audit trail (Tolley et al, 2016). Team members whose ethnic origin differed to mine, assessed whether the interpretations were grounded in the data collected. This allowed me to be conscious of my own bias and subjectivity, and to recognise its distinction from that of the participants.

Results and discussion

Reach

All of the women in the focus groups felt that the programme had successfully reached them, as they had taken part in the majority of events and workshops that were targeted at British African-Caribbean people in the region. They commented positively on marketing and recruitment methods, as this had encouraged them to attend. In particular, all of the women felt that the leaflets advertising the community events and healthy eating workshops were appealing to them, because they included people that 'look like us'. More specifically, they referred to people who can be visually identified as being Black or mixed African-Caribbean. For example, one participant (retired, age 60–65 years) said:

> 'I must commend the leaflets because these people actually look like me and it made me actually look up and think: yes I can attend this.'

Similar comments were made about those members who recruited them or invited them to attend the programme:

> 'I love the leaflets – I can see this lady on the front doing some exercise and that helps to get Caribbean people's attention.' (Community engagement worker – female African-Caribbean, age 55–60 years)

Many of the women felt that the community engagement workers who were of African-Caribbean origin also played an influential role in inviting them to attend. African-Caribbean faith leaders and other members in the community or church group who invited them to attend were also motivational for them. For the majority of the women, this was informed by a lack of distrust towards healthcare professionals who were not African or African-Caribbean. Participants described experiences of racism and ostracism due to their race and/or ethnicity in healthcare settings. These experiences contributed to these shared feelings of marginalisation from healthcare provision among the women, and impacted significantly on many of the women's willingness to access any forms of other NHS-driven services that were not tailored to them. Notably, the following women stated:

> 'When you go to see the GP or nurse, they treat you differently, and it impacts on how Caribbean people feel about other services.' (Female, employed, age 50–55 years).

> 'I don't think the health services and healthy type programmes are there for us, I feel outside of what provide, especially by the staff.' (Female, self-employed, age 40–45 years).

These findings support research that has found that African-Caribbean women who feel unwelcome and marginalised because of their race are less likely to re-enter the health services system or associated provisions (Scott, 2001; Brown et al, 2007; Bhopal, 2012). To address this, all of the women in this research felt that the African-Caribbean people should be representative and included in the recruitment process and delivery. For example, one woman (employed, age 30–35 years) explained:

> 'Sometimes Caribbean people telling other Caribbean people is vital for getting the information around about the

programme, because we have all have been treated in the same way, when you go for check-up or try to join some programme they [the providers] don't understand us, our circumstances, but we listen to others like us.'

For these women, the solution for improving their engagement was not to solely utilise African-Caribbean staff for programme recruitment, but also to ensure that some members of the team were representative of their race and ethnicity as achieved in the programme. For example, one woman explained:

'I was recruited by …, and she's Caribbean. I came because she invited me. I trust her because she's from our [African-Caribbean] community, she knows lots of people I know, but she gets me … and understands the things I have going on with the kids, the caring, work and everything.' (Female, employed, age 40–45 years)

Similar to the research by Noakes (2010), they wanted to have access to other African-Caribbean people who had T2DM or who had successfully reduced their risk or reversed this condition. However, for the women in this research, the gender of this ambassador or champion was important. They also wanted women (African-Caribbean) to take these roles, because they felt they would have a better understanding of the challenges and barriers that women face in looking after their own health – most importantly, the multiple intersecting inequalities they face.

Despite our successes in reaching these women, there were numerous discussions of their shared feelings of being invisible and unheard by clinical commissioners and healthcare providers, because of their gender, race and ethnicity. This was reflected in their discussions of being perceived as hard to reach:

'It frustrates so much when people keep saying we are hard to reach – they all do it in health services. We are not hard to reach, what did we do wrong – we are here, they [service providers] are not coming to us: to understand and know us?'. (Female, employed, age 55–60 years)

These women were agreed that the failure to engage in former services does not lie with them (Edge, 2008, 2013), but with the healthcare providers who misunderstand their differentiated lifestyles and health needs:

> 'We are known as the hard to reach group ... but that is not the case, your [health services] are just not reaching us and understanding our needs as Caribbean people.' (Retired, age 60–65 years)

These women also felt that they were categorised homogeneously as a single group, without recognition that each of their needs are different (Bowleg, 2012; Mwangi and Constance-Huggins, 2017). This is evidenced in the following extract from two of the participants:

> 'We are seen as hard to reach ... because no one has ever actually taken time off, until now, to actually think about us as African-Caribbean people, as actual human beings, we are just a number to them. They just look at us and say a number. They say let's just shut them up and give them this.' (Employed, age 55–60 years)

> 'I don't feel important at all, I think they just see me as another black person and they just push you through as quickly as they can.' (Retired, age 60–65 years).

What was also important within these women's narratives are the intersecting dimensions of differences and marginalisation that relate to their socioeconomic position, geographical locations, age, gender and physical mobility. Discussions of social isolation were common in their narrative, and for some this was interconnected with their rurality. While they recognised that we had successfully managed to reach African-Caribbean women like them who were located in rural villages outside of the city, they commented on the need to keep reaching other women who are also isolated and unable to engage due to other dimensions of intersectionality. This is evidenced in the comments made by three of the women, who discuss the intersections of disability, socioeconomic position and age:

> 'Yes I think that this programme has reached Caribbean people, because some people have come all the way from out of town to come here and attend the events. However, I still think that people attending like us now should be talking to other Caribbean people and women about it,

who are isolated too so that when we do decide to have another meeting, others could come too not just those in the existing groups. We need to get to those who are isolated like I was.' (Employed, age 50–55 years)

'There are people who don't have contact with their children or family and don't have anybody – who are housebound. So targeting them is important, they are also less mobile than me and can't afford taxis here and there.' (Employed, age 35–40 years)

'I'm disabled so I don't know what some of these other services provide … those services and activities don't reach me because I'm housebound and many of them are for men. If it's only a few steps like it has been today, then it's great, but anything else then no … every move I make hurts.' (Retired, age 50–55 years)

Similar to the work of Public Health England (2017), Khan (2012) and Ray and Reed (2005), these BME women felt underrepresented and isolated in rural locations. The intersection of ethnicity and geography is potentially important here for understanding social isolation and health. This is because research suggests that BME people are healthier when they live in areas with a higher concentration of people from their own ethnic group, a so-called 'ethnic density effect' (Halpern and Nazroo, 2000; Pickett and Wilkinson, 2008).

Furthermore, research in the US shows that residence in an area with high black racial isolation is associated with a higher Body Mass Index and higher odds of obesity among women (Chang et al, 2009). The ethnic density effect was identifiable in the comments raised by women in this research who were located in rural locations. They felt that their exclusion from the connection to African-Caribbean communities who were located in the urban areas impacted on their health. Notably, for some women this impacted on their opportunity to engage in lifestyle change programmes that were located in cities, but also to meet with other women from their own ethnic group who would potentially take part in healthy lifestyle activities. For example, one participant explained:

'We don't really have many Black Caribbean people where I live, we do have some black people sometimes, but they are mainly students and they leave. I can walk around, and

I don't see a black face. There are some working in the university, but they leave after studying; one lady who lives near me stayed while she was working there but that is it. We used to walk together sometimes, but now she's left.' (Employed, age 55–60 years)

In addition to rurality, the women's socioeconomic positions impacted on their ability to reach and access the programme. For example, this is reflected in the following comment by one of the women, who also attributed her isolation to the mobility of elder Caribbean people since the Windrush migration period, but also felt that her working hours and lack of finances limited her engagement with former centralised services. She felt that her parents were more socially connected to other African-Caribbean people, because they were geographically located close to other African-Caribbean people who had also newly arrived in the UK:

'They need to recognise we are not all central [living in the urban centre] anymore like when other Caribbean people first came here, most of us will go into town but we all live further out and apart now. When ... our parents came to England everybody was centralised in the city areas, but now we are all over the place. If services are centralised, then that its ok if you can afford to get there, but they [service providers] still do not capture other people like us because we are far away and working longer hours than other women.' (Employed, age 45–50 years)

The majority of these women were working full-time, some of whom were "working two jobs", were on temporary contracts, and were located in roles that included longer than average working hours (female, employed, age 30–35 years). This impacted on the availability to attend structured education or prevention programmes that failed to recognise their working lives.

For example, one participant (age 40–45 years) explained: "with my work shifts and the kids, I'm not able to attend classes and programmes". All of the other women were located in roles (primarily within the public sector) that made them particularly vulnerable to challenges with managing personal health because of their socioeconomic positioning. Some of the women were retired, but also had talked of their socioeconomic positioning and how it differs to that of white British women. Notably, one participant commented:

'Lots of the ladies that I have worked with are already retired and have time to do lots of activities, they play golf and tennis, but they are not African or Caribbean.' (Employed, age 55–60 years)

The majority of the women also commented on the intersections of gender and responsibilities of "caring for your own" that also impacted on their ability to engage with services. For example, one participant commented:

'We Caribbean women care for everyone; we take responsibility for all the family and our parents. I'm caring for my Dad at the moment, he's not well.' (Employed, age 60–65 years)

Despite this, they were all positive about the family-orientated nature of the events that were evidenced in the marketing material that represented African-Caribbean families. The opportunity to bring family members (including children and elder parents, or relatives) was particularly appealing to them. They wanted more opportunities to join lifestyle programmes that recognised their centrality of family, and their cultural practices of sharing responsibility for caring and childrearing. They also wanted providers to recognise that African-Caribbean women specifically contribute to the caring of other family members, and act as beacons in supporting and unifying the family network (Chamberlain, 2003). These women perceived themselves as the most important source of emotional, social and instrumental support within their families, and caring responsibilities were central to their familial roles. They often described themselves as "superwomen", who were responsible for the health of others but had less time to care for themselves – or if they did, they wanted to do this quietly, away from family who could witness their vulnerability:

'As black people, especially women, will always look after our own, we will care for our own or someone in the family will look after that person, so programmes about our diabetes and other health issues need to target us in the right way.' (Employed, age 40–45 years)

The intersection of their socioeconomic positioning also played a role in their ability to be reached when caring for family. For example, one of the women commented on the impact that caring for others with limited finances has on their ability to attend health interventions or programmes:

> 'I have to provide care for my father who actually has diabetes and I help out with childcare for my children because they can't afford it. So, I don't get much time to come to events like this and when I do, I want to be able bring them along ... and it needs to be cheap.' (Employed, age 55–60 years)

What is evident from the women's comments regarding the reach of the programme is that these women feel oppressed and marginalised in their healthcare access, due to the structural and cultural inequalities that include rurality, socioeconomic position, gender and racism. The recruitment and marketing methods that were employed for the programme worked towards addressing the experiences of racism and subsequent mistrust that these women have of healthcare providers. This was because it removed some the challenges they have in accessing and utilising T2DM prevention and management supporting services.

It is important to recognise here the potential consequences that these women may experience as a result of being perceived as invisible and hard to reach in health promotion programmes. Research shows that there is a relationship between marginality and racism experienced by African-Caribbean women and poorer health outcomes (Butler et al, 2002; Heim et al, 2011). As these women perceive themselves as "superwomen", responsible for the health of others as opposed to their own, diabetes prevention and lifestyle change programmes need to include opportunities that extend to all of the Caribbean family, but also to provide activities that recognise the multitude of responsibilities they have – and the interconnected dimensions of intersectionality that impact on their ability to be reached.

Efficacy and adoption

For the women present within the focus groups, the intervention had impacted *effectively* on raising their awareness and prevention of T2DM. This was achieved through the knowledge and activities that focused on increasing physical activity, sitting less and eating more healthily. All of the women also explained that they had *adopted* the programme through their engagement with various activities. They also reported healthy eating and physical activity behaviour changes that had continued beyond the programmes into their daily lives. This is discussed by two of the women in the following extracts:

> 'I have already changed the way I eat as a result of this programme. Since we had that workshops with the dietician lady. I now don't have salt in my food anymore and I've cut down my sugar and occasionally I might have one sugar. So it has benefitted me.' (Employed, age 30–35 years)

> 'I have less sugar since I started the programme ... I have cut out a lot of green banana. I found out from the test [HBa1c] you gave us that I have diabetes, so I don't eat a lot [of green banana] anymore but I found out in the food session that I can have it but not when it's sweet. I've also cut down on the amount of saltfish and now I've only it had it once since I've been here.' (Retired, age 60–65 years)

The culturally tailored physical activities and resources were described by the women as *effective* methods for increasing their physical activity, and for decreasing their sedentary time and their levels of salt, sugar and fat. In particular, the provision of the adapted healthy eating booklets that included traditional Caribbean food and drinks were particularly welcomed by the women. They all commented positively on the culturally specific Eatwell Plate in the booklet that included traditional Caribbean food and drink that were an inherent part of their daily diets (Public Health England, 2018). For example, two of the women explained:

> 'The booklets have helped considerably because they are applicable to our foods.' (Retired, age 65–75 years)

> 'I'm eating different things, I still eat our food, but I do different things with it now. I cook it differently, less oil and more baking.' (Employed, age 50–55 years)

For these women, the programme's healthy eating booklets and workshops addressed the marginality they experienced in health promotion programmes, the NHS and diabetes care. The sessions allowed them to learn alternative ways of cooking the food they consumed, without being encouraged to change to traditional western diets. This supports research by Ochieng (2011), who found that African-Caribbean people feel neglected in messages about healthy diets. As the programme was fully funded, the women welcomed the access to free resources, healthy Caribbean food and guidance from the dieticians, because their socioeconomic status had a strong influence on their ability to change their eating behaviours. They felt that they did not have to balance concerns about healthy eating with those of affordability, particularly because traditional Caribbean foods were provided that they could not otherwise afford. For example, one woman expressed her difficulty in being able to afford to eat healthier Caribbean food:

> 'Traditional Caribbean cooking from scratch has changed because of the price. We are not able to follow the national health promotions, or diets because they don't often use the food we eat but also they are too expensive. We use lots of spinach, fish, aubergine, pumpkin and okra etc. but now it's more expensive. The opportunity to try free food and see the different ways of cooking them has really helped me change how I cook for my family.' (Employed, age 50–55 years)

For these women, culturally tailored and gender-appropriate physical activity sessions had helped them to reduce their risk of T2DM or manage it. The Caribbean Soca carnival workout sessions, yoga, and seated resistance-band exercise and yoga provided opportunities to prevent diabetes, to be active and to manage their weight. Similar to the methods used for marketing and recruitment of the programme, all of the women wanted visible minorities, that being African or African-Caribbean women, not only to deliver the lifestyle change activities, but also to support guidance about diabetes and diabetes risk in BME populations. Similar to the research by Ochieng (2011), these women were more willing to engage in physical activity and lifestyle activities when there were African-Caribbean women who represent them but also offer less Eurocentric activities. The Soca workouts and yoga sessions were particularly enjoyable for the women, because they identified them as being more culturally appropriate. The Soca sessions – Carnival music-based dance classes – gave the participants a chance to dance to a genre that was culturally relevant for them.

Research has shown that culturally specific dance interventions for Black African American women improve health outcomes and functional capacity (Turner et al, 1995). In light of this, these types of programmes are feasible and potentially effective for African-Caribbean women. However, attention must be drawn to the importance of recognising that intersectionality cannot be applied homogeneously to all BME women, by assuming that they all experience similar inequalities (Bowleg, 2012; Mwangi and Constance-Huggins, 2017).

All of the women felt that their knowledge about T2DM and their increased risk had been improved significantly through the programme. One method identified by all of the women as being most successful, was the provision of GPs and nurses at community events. This supports research showing that advice and guidance from a medical professional are motivating for health behaviour change among BME people (Rai and Finch, 1997). However, these women did express the need for representation of visible minorities, as they had encouraged them to "sit up", "pay attention" and actually "do something about it" and act.

All of the women who were present at the focus groups explained that they had *adopted* the programme, some to varying degrees. All of the women attended the first community event targeted at African and African-Caribbean groups. The majority had attended all of the healthy eating workshops, the Soca workout and the seated yoga. However, none of the women had attended the circuit and boxing sessions, and only ten of the women had attended the celebration event. Their level of adoption with the programme activities was impacted by the women's availability, working lives and the relevance of the delivery of activities.

A key influencing factor in their ability to engage was employment and work commitments. As discussed earlier, African-Caribbean women have longer working hours and thus less available time to engage at weekends and in evenings (Breach and Yaojun, 2017). While the programme had sought to provide activities during traditional non-working hours and allowed children to attend (to address potential childcare issues), some women still found it difficult to adopt all of the programme. For example, one woman explained:

> 'I work full-time and weekends, so it was difficult for me to attend all of the group sessions. So we still need activities outside of these times that allow people to attend but also more of the activities that we can do at home or other places.' (Employed, 40–45 years)

The location of the programme delivery was raised a number of times by the women in the six focus groups. The community-based delivery was perceived positively and was important to these women; however, further recommendations were made to provide the programme in additional settings, such as churches and via supported home-based programmes:

> 'I think you've done a great job to get some of the people from the ... [reference made to Christian church with predominantly African-Caribbean congregation] church, but you could do more in the ... [Black] church and some of the African churches.' (Employed, age 50–55 years)

> 'I've really loved coming to this programme, but I think there could be some more resources to allow us to do it at home, especially when we can't get out.' (Retired, age 60–65 years)

As discussed by Brown et al (2007), religion and faith play an important role in guiding African-Caribbean people's daily lives, and are influential to the perceptions they have about diabetes, diabetes risk and associated lifestyle practices. Elsewhere, it has been evidenced that religious beliefs or faith can impact on African-Caribbean women's adoption of health promotion and diabetes programmes (Higginbottom, 2006) and they can feature as a dimensions of minority women's intersectionality (Reimer-Kirkham and Sharma, 2011). However, for these women, the church can assist in improving health outcomes. In the US, churches and other faith organisations are increasingly popular settings in which to conduct health promotion and diabetes prevention programmes for African American women (McNabb et al, 1997; Young and Stewart, 2006; Bopp et al, 2007; Yanek et al, 2016).

It is recommended here that church-based delivery could be utilised in the UK, but with community-based diabetes prevention programmes. In this programme, churches were attended to facilitate recruitment and faith leaders assisted in recruitment, but church-based delivery could be more effective in improving more consistent adoption for some of the women. Additionally, home-based monitoring interventions that promote physical activity could easily be coupled with the programme, to acknowledge the differentiated working hours that these women may experience.

Research shows that this type of delivery is more broadly accessible and addresses specific barriers that prevent individuals with diabetes and those at risk from participating in physical activity (Agurs-Collins et al, 1997; Mori et al, 2011). The 'Healthier You: NHS Diabetes Prevention Programme' in the UK offers digital supported interventions that include an online app with access to health monitoring, peer support groups and health coaches. This approach is potentially useful for these women. However, if it is to be adopted, the intersections of difference that impact on these women's ability to adopt a programme would also need to be further considered. For example, research elsewhere shows that disability, socioeconomic position of the women and cost of accessing the programme play influential intersecting roles in African American women's engagement in home-based health interventions (Rimmer et al, 2000).

Implementation and maintenance

Many of the women felt that the programme was *implemented* successfully and could be maintained if it were to continue. They expressed feelings of satisfaction that the programme adhered to the intended aims. Despite this, three of the women in one of the focus groups expressed dissatisfaction with the delivery of the final community celebration event and felt that the programme could not be *maintained* if these types of events were to be continued. Due to problems with the venue availability, the event was delivered at a venue in which a Healthy Family Fun Day was being already hosted by a different organisation. While the community event and a Healthy Family Fun Day were two separate events, the women felt that some of the health promotion messages about reducing the risk of T2DM were overshadowed by this family fun day. This was because the other organisation hosted stalls at which candyfloss and fast food were provided. This led to confusion about the intended messages of the programme. For example, two commented:

> 'I liked all the events, but I wasn't so sure about the last event because of the candyfloss and burgers. I liked the seated exercises that we got to do, the free resistance bands and pedometers but the other event being there confused me slightly.' (Employed, age 45–50 years)

> 'Yeh I really like the programme, I definitely feel that I've a lot about how to do more activity and eat less sugar and salt, but I think it that last event could have been hosted at a different time to the other event.' (Retired, age 65–70 years)

For the programme to be *maintained* at individual and community levels, all the women felt that the following needed to be continued in the programme: culturally relevant physical activity and healthy eating activities delivered in community settings; continued recognition of the intersection of oppressions of marginality to be addressed in timing, delivery type and location of delivery; the presence of visible minorities, including African-Caribbean women in all stages of planning, design, delivery and maintenance.

The women felt that the use of community champions from their own communities should assist in maintaining the programme. Notably, two of the women were keen to volunteer themselves, to assist in running parts of the programme and in recruiting other women like them. They felt they should be responsible for their own health and address perceptions of being hard to reach by health services:

> 'I'm really passionate about telling other women about this programme, I think I can help to get other women to come but also support to keep it going. This would make people see that we are here!!' (Employed, 40–45 years)

> 'I actually invited three of the women in the programme to come, so I'd love to learn more and help to get more programmes like this for us.' (Employed, age 50–55 years)

Conclusion

This research has shown that culturally tailored lifestyle behavioural change programmes in community-based locations can help to raise awareness of T2DM for African-Caribbean women. Therefore, these women are not or hard to reach for the delivery of lifestyle behavioural change programmes, but rather are perceived as invisible and therefore the delivery and implementation of programmes do not reach them. To address their perceived invisibility, an intersectional lens is required for creating accessible and effective programmes for these women. Health evaluation frameworks should therefore focus on the interconnected ways in which gender, race and ethnicity and socioeconomic status and other dimensions of marginality impact on British African-Caribbean women's access to diabetes awareness, prevention and management programmes.

For these women, healthy eating and physical activity behaviour changes occur for them when health interventions recognise their different socioeconomic positioning and the interconnected social and cultural barriers they face that prevent them from accessing lifestyle behaviour change programmes. Engagement in lifestyle change programmes, and successful maintenance of healthy eating and weight management, can be enhanced when interventions include culturally tailored marketing, recruitment and delivery strategies. Similar to other evaluation research completed on health interventions with African American women, these programmes should offer women the opportunity to access staff, GPs and community ambassadors who are representative of and understand them. Ideally, these should include women who are of the same ethnic origin and/or thus understand their multidimensional marginality.

Although common barriers to accessing health interventions for minority women include their gender, race and socioeconomic status, this study has shown that additional interconnected barriers exist. What is unique to this study is that other dimensions, including rurality, should be recognised in lifestyle change programme design and delivery for African-Caribbean women. While it was evident in existing intersectionality literature that religion and/or faith can also marginalise minority women (Reimer-Kirkham and Sharma, 2011) from their access to diabetes healthcare and diabetes interventions (Scott, 2001; Brown et al, 2007), here it is evident that church-based delivery and church leaders and/or members are beneficial for improving these women's access to, and adoption of, the programme.

By listening to the voices of African-Caribbean women, clinical commissioners and service providers can do much more – across health promotion and in healthcare provision – to provide resources that are culturally sensitive and accessible. Further understanding of the multidimensional and interconnected inequalities experienced not only by African-Caribbean women but also by other BME women, can assist in improving policy and practice that promotes equality and equity in healthcare access.

Awareness of diabetes risk and lifestyle and dietary behaviour practices can potentially improve for these women, when they have the opportunity to access affordable and accessible activities and are therefore not treated as being hard to reach. The limitations of the programme raised by women here, indicate that community-based, multi-sited places of delivery should be offered by practitioners and/ or researchers. This would allow African-Caribbean women further opportunities to sustain their effective adoption of similar programmes and associated lifestyle behaviour change.

6

South Asian and BME migrant women's experiences of culturally tailored, women-only physical activity programme for improving participation, social isolation and wellbeing

This chapter discusses the delivery and evaluation of a women-only physical activity and yoga programme, designed to improve physical activity levels, social isolation and wellbeing among South Asian and Black and Minority Ethnic (BME) migrant women living in areas of high economic deprivation. The chapter provides an accessible insight into the aims, objectives, methods and findings of the study.

It provides important recommendations on how researchers and service providers can deliver culturally tailored, community-based health interventions, and how an approach to sustainable, community-based interventions can be devised through this type of research. It demonstrates that social support – such as childcare provision, child-friendly sessions and social media forums determined by the target population – can mitigate misconceptions about South Asian and BME migrant women being hard to reach and difficult to engage in physical activity health interventions.

Project and background

The purpose of this project was to deliver a women-only physical activity and yoga programme over a 12-month period. It sought to improve physical activity participation levels, social isolation and wellbeing among South Asian women living in an area of high economic deprivation within an East Midlands city. The programme was targeted at South Asian women, but also attracted Black and Minority Ethnic (BME) migrant women.

It is important here to outline the overlap that commonly occurs between populations belonging to BME and migrant groups. This is because these terms can become conflated, and thus the experiences of ethnicity, race, health and social isolation between the groups can become homogenised. However, these experiences can differ between these groups. BME groups include established minorities as well as those resulting from recent migratory waves. 'Migrants and their descendants, sometimes termed [new arrivals], and second or third generation migrants, often become part of BME communities' (Llácer et al, 2007).

In this study, the South Asian women included women who were born in the UK or who had migrated within the last 10–30 years from Bangladesh. The BME migrant women who participated had migrated within the last 12 months and self-defined themselves as Indian, Arabian and Muslim. Their countries of original residence included India, Italy and Arab countries.

South Asian ethnic minorities, commonly defined as of Indian, Pakistani, Bangladeshi and Sri Lankan origin, are the largest UK ethnic minority group, and display higher rates of lifestyle-related chronic diseases such as Type 2 diabetes (T2DM), cardiovascular disease and obesity compared to white Europeans (Wolf et al, 2020). It is widely known that a physically inactive lifestyle promotes these chronic health conditions. However, South Asian women are underrepresented in terms of their engagement in physical activity. The UK Active Lives Survey (2017/18) highlights that only 50% of South Asian women meet government recommendations of 150 minutes of weekly moderate to vigorous physical activity. As decreased physical fitness is one of the strongest predictors of mortality, it is important to try and implement methods to effectively support this group to ease disease burdens.

South Asian women face specific cultural barriers to physical activity, such as perceived 'appropriateness' of traditional physical activity modalities and the need to be active in female–only spaces (Babakus and Thompson, 2012). South Asian women from certain religious groups have described a sense of otherness and not belonging as they have tried to exercise in public domains. Muslim women, in particular, have experienced verbal abuse and difficulties related to their dress code of mode modesty and the physical presence and gaze of men that has made it difficult for them to participate in physical activity (Whitten and Thompson, 2005). South Asian women living in areas of high economic deprivation can also experience additional socioeconomic barriers in accessing physical activity. This can be accompanied with social isolation due to parental responsibilities and household tasks, or cultural norms surrounding mixed-gender activities. These can promote anxiety and stress (Karasz et al, 2019) and can be responsible for the elevated levels of depression observed in South Asian women (Razieh et al, 2019).

BME migrant women living in the UK are also reported to have a higher level of obesity and are less physically active than white Europeans (Lawton et al, 2006). However, insufficient attention has been paid to understanding their health and physical activity needs, resulting in the growth of health inequalities among BME female migrants. They have disproportionately higher rates of mortality when compared to the host population. Therefore, physical activity interventions are needed to assist in easing disease burdens and improving health status. New arrivals are at risk of being unable to access physical activity interventions when they arrive in a host nation, because of their socioeconomic position, cultural beliefs regarding physical activity, deprivation and lack of access to services (Visram et al, 2007; Khanam and Costarelli, 2008; Caperchione et al, 2009). They are also more vulnerable to social isolation because of their cultural beliefs, family responsibilities and financial positioning (Sriskantharajah and Kai, 2007). There are misperceptions about the specific health needs of migrants, due to poor communication between public health services and limited understanding about how to deliver culturally relevant services. The situation is compounded by the problems that migrants face in accessing health and wellbeing services. This can result in these groups being perceived as hard to reach by researchers and health providers.

Previous research has shown that access to women-only physical activity programmes can play a significant role in increasing the health and wellbeing of the South Asian and BME migrant women. The health benefits include reducing the risk of many chronic conditions, such as T2DM, coronary heart disease, obesity and many mental health conditions (Hayes et al, 2002; Babakus and Thompson, 2012). Research also shows that they can be successfully engaged when strategies are culturally appropriate and tailored to and for them. Culturally relevant physical activity opportunities for South Asian and BME migrant women, such as yoga, can help to address barriers that prevent access and participation (Rizzolo et al, 2020). Yoga is a form of physical activity that is informed by an Indian wellbeing system comprising physical movements, meditation and breathing exercises, and is a practice that is linked to cultural beliefs within some South Asian communities (Sengupta, 2012). Over recent years, yoga has become increasingly prominent in improving physical and mental wellbeing worldwide. However, as with other modes of physical activity, yoga is not always accessible to South Asian and BME migrant women in the UK, due to location of delivery and a lack of culturally and/or religiously appropriate public recreational provision and facilities However, this form of activity is accessible for a multi-ethnic population.

Yoga has been reported to improve health in addition to prevention and management of chronic conditions. Specifically, research in yoga has shown that it positively affects mental wellbeing, hypertension, obesity, T2DM and physical fitness (Sengupta, 2012; Tenfelde et al, 2018). South Asian and BME migrant women are at increased risk of developing such conditions, therefore the potential effects of yoga reducing the risks are relevant. Additionally, BME migrant and South Asian women are at increased risk of depression and anxiety (Husain et al, 2012), therefore understanding whether weekly physical activity and yoga sessions could improve mental wellbeing in this at-risk population would be particularly important.

Aims and objectives

This study evaluated delivery of weekly yoga sessions alongside physical activity sessions for South Asian and BME migrant women at a community cultural centre. Notable knowledge gaps that this study sought to fill include: the acceptability and accessibility of a yoga and physical activity programmes in BME migrant and South Asian women; and the impact that such activity programmes have on social isolation and mental wellbeing. Therefore, the specific aims of this research were to:

• examine the level of participation in a 30-week, community-based physical activity programme that includes yoga and exercise classes for South Asian women and BME migrant women aged 18 years and above;
• gain insight into the effectiveness of the physical activity programme on improving South Asian women's access to, and participation in, physical activity through focus groups with the participants;
• investigate the South Asian and BME migrant women's experiences of the sessions and the impact on their self-reported social isolation and wellbeing.

The objectives of the research were to:

• complete attendance surveys to record women's level of participation in a women-only physical activity (yoga and exercise classes) programme delivered over a period of one year (30 weeks);

- complete focus groups to qualitatively measure whether those delivering the programme and its participants perceive that the physical activity programme improves BME migrant and South Asian women's access to, and participation in, physical activity;
- complete focus groups, to qualitatively measure BME migrant and South Asian women's experiences of the sessions and the impact on their social isolation and wellbeing.

Programme evaluation

The women-only yoga and physical activity programme was delivered at a Bangladeshi cultural community organisation, located within an economically deprived ward in an East Midlands city, with a diverse BME population. The programme was advertised by the community organisation and the BME female community research team to South Asian women aged 18 years and above, living within the local community. The programme offered two one-hour physical activity sessions (aerobic sessions and yoga) per week for a duration of 30 weeks[1] over a period of one year. The specific type of yoga delivered was Vinyasa Flow yoga, including mediation and breathing exercises. These sessions were delivered by BME female qualified fitness and yoga instructor.

Ten health awareness sessions on culturally relevant healthy eating practices were also delivered alongside this programme by female South Asian trained demonstrators, who were employed at the community organisation, and by residents in the local community. The programme allowed women to be accompanied by their children, who were offered peer childcare support during their participation in the programme.

Methods

This evaluation measured BME migrant and South Asian women's uptake of the women-only yoga and physical activity programme via attendance records at the start and at 12 months. Five focus groups (of one–two hours) were arranged at the end of the project, where the participants could discuss the physical activity programme. This allowed for a qualitative insight into the uptake of the programme, as well as other important perceptions of the programme regarding physical activity levels, social isolation and wellbeing.

---

[1] This excluded school holidays, during which the centre and crèche facilities were closed.

Prior to the physical activity programme beginning, participants were asked to complete a self-reported physical activity questionnaire (IPAQ – Short Form), which assessed the types and intensity of physical activity and sitting time that people do as part of their daily lives, to estimate total Physical Activity in MET-min/week and time spent sitting (Cora et al, 2003). The participants were provided with support to complete these forms by the female researcher and the female South Asian community worker. Similarly, at the end of the 12-month physical activity programme, participants were invited to complete this questionnaire.

Provisions were made available for any individuals who did not understand any aspects of the questions in this questionnaire and interview (via members of community centre staff who were translators). All qualitative data gathered was audio recorded, transcribed, anonymised and subsequently deleted, protecting the identity of the participants. A thematic analysis of data was completed.

Evaluation findings

South Asian women's level of participation

A total of 83 women (between the ages of 18 and 55 years and over) who migrated to the UK or were UK-born but whose parents are foreign-born or foreign nationals, joined the programme (see Table 6.1).

The programme was most popular among women between the ages of 26 and 45 years. The women self-identified as:

- Bangladeshi (n=57)
- Indian (n=6)
- Arabian (n=17)
- White/Muslim (n=3).

The majority of the women did not have long-term health conditions. However, all of the women described themselves as being overweight or obese, and some reported conditions including T2DM, arthritis, asthma, anxiety and low mood. The yoga and physical activity aerobic sessions were attended by women only, as advertised. However, wider family members accompanied women to the healthy eating workshops, including husbands and children. The yoga and physical activity sessions were enjoyed by all of the women, but were most popular among women between the ages of 26 and 45 years (73%).

Table 6.1: Participation data

Yoga and aerobic sessions	Age range	Gender		Ethnicity			
		F		Bangladeshi	Indian	Arabian	White/Muslim
		43 (Total)		32	4	6	1
	18–25	1					
	26–35	18					
	36–45	15					
	46–55	6					
	55 and over	3					
Healthy Eating workshops		M	F	Bangladeshi	Indian	Arab	White/Muslim
		11	33	29	2	11	2
	18–25		5				
	26–35		13				
	36–45		21				
	46–55		4				
	55 and over		1				

Effectiveness of the programme in improving women's access to, and participation in, physical activity

All of the women scored a LOW level of physical activity on the IPAQ completed at the start of the project. None of these women were meeting any of the criteria for either MODERATE or HIGH levels of physical activity per week. The IPAQ revealed that their activity centred primarily on domestic commitments as part of managing their house/home and family.

Completion of the IPAQ data at the end of the project showed that the women were completing MODERATE levels of physical activity per week. The women's self-reported comments on physical activity levels made during the interviews supported this, as all of the women had increased their physical activity levels since participating in the programme. For example, the following comments were made by women attending the programme:

> 'I've been attending at least every week.'
> 'I make sure I come every week.'
> 'I've come every week but only on the Tuesday sessions.'

Many of the women also felt that the programme had encouraged them to participate in physical activity (yoga and aerobics) at home, either independently or with wider family members. For example, the following women commented:

> 'I started doing the yoga and Zumba at home with my husband and daughter, actually I was doing it at home and then my husband and daughter joined in.'

> 'I have aches and pains so now when I get them, I try and do some yoga exercises at home to help.'

> 'I've been doing the plan and tummy exercises at home.'

> 'The neck exercises we do are good for me when I'm breast feeding, so I do them at home too.'

All of the women felt that the programme had been effective in improving their access to physical activity through the provision of women-only sessions. None of the women had taken part in yoga or aerobic sessions prior to the programme, as the majority of them had previously experienced difficulties in accessing exercise classes and wider physical activity, due to the provision of mixed-gender sessions and male instructors.

These findings support research by Whitten and Thompson (2005), in which religious and/or cultural beliefs prevented Muslim women from exercising in public domains due to the lack of women-only spaces and the dominated physical presence and gaze of men. These barriers, and how they have been addressed through the programme, are discussed in the following comments by five of the women:

> 'At the main gym in town, they have an area for women to go in the gym, but they don't have women only exercises classes, or women instructors so I can't go. I really wanted to join but what's the point when you can't join the classes.'

'I feel comfortable here, I'm now doing a lot more because it's comfortable here, and you can exercise without worrying.'

'It's enjoyable here because like normally you try go to like the local gym and it was mixed classes so you couldn't do Pilates or anything.'

'I don't feel embarrassed here to take part ... I feel more comfortable.'

'I've only experienced programmes like this for women back at home in Italy, but nothing here.'

Experiences of the sessions and the impact on social isolation and wellbeing

Women's discussions about their experiences of the sessions indicated that there had been health benefits, notably to their physical and mental health. Predominantly, participants highlighted the benefits of yoga and aerobics sessions as being fun, enjoyable, and good for their weight loss, energy, mind and health. For example, the following four participants explained:

'I love the aerobic sessions it's fun and enjoyable.'

'I feel like I have more energy from doing the sessions.'

'I've managed to lose weight doing this programme and I feel so much more confident.'

'I definitely feel happier since taking part.'

'I feel calmer ... it takes me away from the stress and commitments at home.'

The women also commented on the impact of the sessions in improving existing mobility and medical conditions, such as arthritis, asthma and stress. This was explained by three participants:

'I feel fewer aches and pains from the classes and I'm more mobile.'

'Yoga has been helpful because I got asthma and it helped me a lot thinking about your breathing and it makes you relax more.'

'I've got a lot in my mind, so the classes have helped me a lot to clear my mind.'

The overall impact of the programme on their social isolation was described by all of the women as positive. A number of the women commented on how the programme had "got [them] out of the house" and allowed them to "meet other women they wouldn't normally meet". Importantly, four women also commented on the opportunities it offered for them to integrate with people from other countries and women who are new arrivals to the UK:

'I've met other women from different communities beyond the Bangladeshis.'

'It opens us up to meet people from other cultures.'

'You get to meet more people here and to integrate with people who have been in the UK longer than us.'

'It's such a diverse community as well like you meet so many different people ... everybody together is better.'

The women also aligned this new interaction with others as being beneficial to their own wellbeing and mental health. For example, the following participant explained:

'It's good for us to meet other people, for our health, meeting people, because it's good for the social interaction.'

One of the central benefits of the programme for the women was the provision of crèche facilities. All of the women had childcare responsibilities for their own children or their family member's children. This impacted on their opportunity to socialise and exercise. As the community organisation provided space for children to attend, the women felt that the programme addressed their social isolation and the barriers they faced in accessing exercise.

Migrant women and women from BME backgrounds can face particular risks of social isolation because they experience greater socioeconomic disadvantages, for example poverty, poor housing and unemployment (Llácer et al, 2007). All of the women in this study experienced these difficulties, because they resided in an inner-city area characterised by high economic deprivation, high unemployment, poverty and poor-quality public spaces. Furthermore, some of the women, who were new arrivals to the UK, were experiencing marginalisation processes and structures linked to their migrant ethnic identities. For example, some were experiencing financial difficulties, because they were unable to access employment or speak English, and this impacted on their opportunity to join social activities, access childcare and meet other people.

These barriers can hamper the development of social networks and enhance social isolation for new migrants to the UK (McCabe et al, 2013). However, the provision of bilingual staff and free access to the programme allowed the women to participate and improve their wellbeing and social isolation. For example, two of the migrant women discussed the benefits:

> 'I only came here a few months ago. I can't get work yet and I have just been at home and lonely. My husband works all the time and we can't afford to pay for nursery or anything. This programme has been great for me mentally and physically because I can bring the children … I have met many other ladies and it's helping me to lose weight.'

> 'It's nice here because there are other women who speak [my language] Arabic. I've also been able to get out of the house with my children. I've been stuck at home since arrived and it's been really difficult … you know mentally and emotionally … especially being in a new country where you don't know anyone.'

Limitations and recommendations for researchers and practitioners

While the programme has been beneficial to the women's health, wellbeing and social isolation, there were limitations in its delivery. Notably, the timing, frequency and delivery of physical activities could have been improved to enhance the women's sustained participation in the programme. It was recommended by both staff members and some of the participants that the aerobic and yoga sessions should be delivered consecutively on the same day. These sessions were delivered on different days during the week. Furthermore, all of the women requested for the sessions to be held more frequently.

While it has been reported that South Asian and BME migrant women experience social isolation (Sriskantharajah and Kai, 2007), the level of social isolation that these women experience was far greater than anticipated. They expressed a greater demand for accessible health and physical interventions such as these. Recommendations here would be to: increase the number of sessions available; and include supplementary opportunities for the women to interact and socialise with other women that adhere to their cultural practices and traditions.

Evaluation of the programme could also be developed to improve monitoring of the women's physical activity and sedentary behaviour during and at the end of the programme. For example, the IPAQ short form questionnaire could have been administrated more frequently at three and/or six months. Also, researchers and practitioners could provide participants with additional options to complete the form over the telephone or virtually at the end of the project, with the provision of translation, to enhance completion rates.

While the programme had been designed in collaboration with BME women to avoid religious and cultural festivals, prayers and related activities, some of the participants were unable to complete the IPAQ at the end of the programme, due to these types of commitments. Therefore, it is recommended that researchers or providers talk to their participants further at the start of the programme, about any additional religious or cultural commitments they may have that will impact on the evaluation.

While, it is evident that the IPAQ is available in different languages, and the meaning of the words have been adapted for different ethnic populations and country contexts (Tran et al, 2020), the cultural relevance of the survey has not been developed – and it was not culturally relevant for these women. Therefore, the cultural relevance and/or appropriateness of the IPAQ should be developed for further research with BME migrant and South Asian women. Studies have been completed to assess the interpretation of specific questions and the relevance of the concepts to Latino communities in the US (Arredondo et al, 2012). However, this could be developed further in the UK, and supported with qualitative research to understand different forms of participation in physical activity among BME migrant and South Asian women.

For researchers interested in more clinical and accurate tracking of physical activity participation than self-reported accounts, this evaluation could be extended with the use of accelerometers or Fitbit devices. However, it is recommended that the provision of translation and female research staff should be included, to support the women's use of these devices. Further qualitative work should also be completed to ascertain the acceptability of use.

The provision of childcare was identified as being essential for the women's ability to participate in the sessions. As these women were located in areas of high economic deprivation and were positioned in low socioeconomic positions, funding is needed to provide sustained crèche support for mothers attending the sessions. This assisted in increasing uptake and sustained participation for the duration of the programme. However, it is important to recognise that this programme was delivered in a community-based venue that was accessible to them and was perceived by the women as being a culturally appropriate space. Notably, the community-based venue offered the women rooms in which to pray and access to childcare staff who spoke their languages and were accustomed to their cultural and religious practices. As the staff were valued, it was also recommended that they could assist in providing children's physical activity and yoga sessions for older children alongside the current activities in these venues.

While the programme activities and childcare provision improved the emotional wellbeing and social isolation of the women, recommendations were made by them and by staff to make further use of social media such as WhatsApp. The women commonly used WhatsApp as a method for connecting with family and friends within their own BME communities. They valued its use as a method for recruitment and notification tool by the BME female community staff member. However, they also wanted to develop their own WhatsApp group to connect with other women and offer social networking opportunities beyond the face-to-face sessions. Therefore, it is recommended that researchers and practitioners utilise these tools with BME women in intervention delivery. However, it should be noted that other forms of social media that are commonly utilised by healthcare providers, organisations and research bodies, such as Twitter, were not valued by the women.

Conclusion

This programme has successfully increased the uptake of South Asian and BME migrant women taking part in a physical activity programme. The collected data indicates effectiveness of the programme, as there were self-reported increases in physical activity participation levels among the majority of the women.

Furthermore, the qualitative data indicates that the women participating in the programme experienced improved wellbeing and reduced social isolation. This data also illustrates that some women experienced improved self-confidence to participate in physical activity beyond the project, notably via home practice with wider family.

Recommendations for future delivery should continue to recognise the culturally relevant programme design (for example, South Asian and BME migrant women-only sessions, culturally relevant activities, and delivery in culturally relevant community venues). Furthermore, it should be recognised that social support, such as providing childcare, child-friendly sessions and social media forums, as determined by the target population, can mitigate barriers to participation among South Asian and BME women.

Evaluation of these types of programmes could be developed by further monitoring of women's physical activity by cultural training research and/or BME community members to support in delivery of the IPAQ form and use of accelerometers. If the IPAQ is to be utilised, it should be culturally adapted with the support of South Asian and BME migrant women. Further focus groups and interviews with these women could also improve comprehension, interpretation, and the cultural relevance of the physical activity questions to these women.

7

Experiences of health and wellbeing during periods of fragile and uncertain citizenship among African-Caribbean migrant groups

According to the most recent figures, there are approximately 594,825 Black African-Caribbean people in England and Wales, making up 1.1% of the total population (Office for National Statistics, 2011). The UK African-Caribbean population includes migrants originating from various Caribbean islands. However, many of these migrants in the UK have experienced differentiated experiences in health and wellbeing since their migration from the West Indies. Immigration policies, experiences of marginalisation and racism, and inequalities in access to healthcare have contributed to their poorer health outcomes. The UK hostile environment policy, in particular, has created an atmosphere of fear among these individuals and has deterred some from seeking healthcare (NHS England, 2019; Weller et al, 2019). Beyond this, those who have moved from the West Indies, have – and continue to be impacted by – experiences of racism, marginalisation and fragile citizenship or uncertain residency status; these have impacted significantly on their health and wellbeing and that of their family members (Chouhan and Nazroo, 2020).

This chapter draws on research that explores the existing impact of migration and uncertain residency on the health and wellbeing of African-Caribbean heritage communities. The chapter outlines how participants of African-Caribbean heritage experience their health, wellbeing and healthcare access since their arrival in the UK and during periods of fragile and uncertain citizenship.

This chapter also includes an exploration of the risks for the wellbeing of existing residents whose migrant status has become uncertain. Life storytelling methods are utilised, to produce bibliographic accounts of the participants who moved to the UK at any time from the 1940s to the present day, or whose immediate family did so. Methods for developing and building sustained partnerships between migrant community members and researchers are also discussed. Specifically, the chapter draws attention to the ways in which future research can be delivered in collaboration with BME migrants, to understand their migration journeys.

The 'Windrush generation' and migration from the West Indies

The 'Windrush group' or 'Windrush generation' are terms commonly used to refer to a group of African-Caribbean people and their descendants who migrated from the West Indies from the 1940s. While the term 'Windrush' is commonly used in reference to those migrants who have moved from the West Indies up to the present day, it actually refers to the name of the ship, the SS Empire Windrush, that brought the mass migration of people from the Caribbean islands to Tilbury Docks in Britain on 22 June 1948 (Goff, 2019).

Although migration of African-Caribbean people to the UK had existed prior to this (Sutherland, 2006; Peplow, 2020), the political rationale for mass migration at this time was to help rebuild the employment and transport infrastructure that had suffered after the Second World War (Taylor, 2018). Migrants on this ship were primarily from the Caribbean Islands within the West Indies, such as Jamaica and Trinidad, but there were also migrants and refugees from other countries.

African-Caribbean people who have migrated from the West Indies since this period have been impacted by experiences of racism, fragile citizenship or uncertain residency status (Chouhan and Nazroo, 2020). This has been impacted by the development of aggressive immigration policies, notably the hostile environment policy.

Policy impact: hostile environment and migrant status

The hostile environment policy was developed in 2012 by Theresa May, then the Conservative government home secretary. The central aim was to reduce net migration in the UK. Specifically, May sought to reduce the number of people within the UK who were perceived to be here illegally (Arnott, 2019). To achieve this, she created the policy requiring everyone to provide documents confirming their right to be in the country, and their entitlement to access public services or to get a job or rent accommodation (Cole, 2020). This policy differed to former migration policies, because it now required people to meet the burden of proof, thus requiring original documentation. However, to meet the deportation targets May had imposed, officials focused more on denying someone a right to remain. The policy, for some, has resulted in: in-country checks of immigration status, and restricted access to entitlements such as healthcare, social care, housing, benefits and employment (Goodfellow, 2019). Although it remains the case that everybody living in the UK has the legal right to access primary care, one feature of this policy has been the restriction of access to secondary healthcare for visitors; other unintended consequences of this include limited access to registering with a general practitioner (Glennerster and Hodson, 2020).

This policy has been an area of increased public concern, because the inherent focus on meeting the deportation targets has resulted in a number of African-Caribbean people being deported to the West Indies by the UK government. Some, who arrived as children, travelling on their parents' passports, have never applied for travel or citizenship documents, and have been deported to the original home of their parents, their wider family or deceased family members. Others have been returned to their places of birth, many years after they arrived, with little knowledge or understanding of the culture or lifestyle, and no access to a home.

These actions have been referred to publicly as the 'Windrush scandal' of 2018, because it sheds light on unethical Home Office practices, and has been linked to the aggressive compliance environment policy in the Immigration Act 2014 and the Immigration Act 2016 (Cole, 2020). Through the implementation of these Acts, the hostile environment policy included requirements for landlords, and organisations such as the NHS, to carry out ID checks to prove the status and rights, despite their being granted a legal right to live in the country as members of the Commonwealth under the Immigration Act 1972. Specifically, this Act also removed protection for Commonwealth citizens, who had up until then been exempt from deportation. As a result, some citizen-migrants who had entered legally and had had the right to reside in the UK prior to 1972, have been detained or deported (Taylor, 2018).

The UK government has been forced to apologise for wrongfully deporting people and has offered financial compensation for anyone who has suffered loss via the Windrush Compensation Scheme (Gentleman, 2019). However, the UK government and Home Office have received increased criticism, because there have been issues in identifying those who have the right to remain. This is because in 2010, under the Conservative government, the UK Border Force destroyed thousands of landing cards or registry slips that were the only proof of exactly when some migrants arrived in Britain (Goodfellow,

2019). They also neglected to issue migrants with any paperwork to confirm their new status (BBC, 2018). The introduction of the hostile environment policy has created further uncertainty in residency, because without this policy those who moved to the UK prior to 1972 would not have to provide proof of their arrival and legal right to stay. Had they not been destroyed, the landing cards could now be used alongside other documents, to help someone threatened with deportation to build their case for staying. This is, therefore, another contributing factor to the 'Windrush scandal'.

The Home Office has also been criticised for this policy because it has been unable to monitor the overall impact of the policy on the mental and physical health of migrants (Vernon, 2019). Furthermore, the policy measures have caused racism and discrimination in various sectors of society for the Windrush generation and their descendants. Unfortunately, it is unclear how many people have been affected directly and indirectly. Reports continue to come in from the Windrush Taskforce, from researchers and from public media commentators on the people who have been impacted. Given that over 15,000 people have been reported to have migrated from just one of the islands, Jamaica, since 1972, the figures of all those impacted across the islands will not be evident until claims are made and more research is completed (Taylor, 2018).

It is important to recognise that many African-Caribbean people who have been granted residency since moving to the UK from the 1940s have still experienced inequalities in accessing their residency status and healthcare, and often describe feeling out of place and marginalised. Some argue that this has been heightened by African-Caribbean migrants being problematised in public media (Grant, 2019) and public discourse, and categorised by the Immigration and Colonial Office as unwanted outsiders who were less deserving of being members of the existing British society (Sutherland, 2006; Griffiths, 2021). It has been suggested that this experience of being a migrant has also impacted on the health and wellbeing of African-Caribbean people in the form of differentiated health outcomes and inequalities in access to healthcare services.

Migration status and impact on health and wellbeing

Research evidence examining health patterns of African-Caribbean migrants has shown that there are higher rates of chronic health conditions (heart disease, hypertension, diabetes, stroke, arthritis, and any cardiovascular disease or metabolic condition) compared with those left behind at home Caribbean countries (Lacey et al, 2019). Research also shows that mental health conditions, such as dementia, depression and schizophrenia, are markedly higher for African-Caribbean people who have migrated to the UK from the Caribbean than those who have remained in their country of origin (Harrison et al, 1988; Chakraborty and McKenzie, 2012).

As discussed in Chapter 2, differential experiences of racism across sectors of society, and inequalities in access to treatment and detention services among African-Caribbean groups, have played a contributory role in health outcomes. However, while there are multiple risk factors for the higher rates of poor health conditions among African-Caribbean groups, the impact of migration experiences (including racism and uncertain residency) can play a significant role (Wray and Bartholomew, 2006). More recently, there have been urgent calls for mental health and wellbeing programmes on the post-traumatic impact of the hostile environment on the Windrush generation and their descendants (Vernon, 2019). Recommendations for recovery of post-traumatic stress have included culturally tailored support and healing spaces – such as Emotional Emancipation Circles or healing circles (Grills et al, 2016; Vernon, 2019). However, at the time of writing, these programmes have yet to be developed. What has been recognised is that the health and wellbeing of African-Caribbean people who migrated to the UK have experienced differences in their health outcomes, when compared to those in their home country. Questions are therefore often raised as to whether the migration experiences and uncertain residency status have been influential in the health and wellbeing of Caribbean migrants (Wray and Bartholomew, 2006).

Unfortunately, research evidence that captures health outcomes by migration status (for example country of birth, duration of residence, nature of migration status) for African-Caribbean groups in the UK is relatively limited (Bhopal, 2014). While mortality data (death registration) in the UK is according to country of birth, incidence and prevalence data is by ethnicity, which makes it difficult to understand patterns for non-communicable health conditions (for example diabetes, and heart disease and stroke) among migrants (Jayaweera, 2014). Furthermore, a lack of inclusion and standardisation in the conceptualisation and categorisation of migration status in health research and routine administrative health systems also complicates our access to health information and understanding of migration experiences (Jayaweera, 2014; Bhopal, 2014).

Therefore, research that examines the impact of migration status on the health and wellbeing from the perspectives of those who have lived these experiences, can be important in widening our understanding of the injustices that may occur in migration. This research sought to achieve this. Specifically, the aim of this research was to explore how people of African-Caribbean heritage experience their health, wellbeing and healthcare access since their arrival to the UK and during periods of fragile citizenship or uncertain residency such as the hostile environment. The following objectives were set to fulfil this aim:

- to examine the lived experiences of health and wellbeing from the perspectives of people of African-Caribbean heritage who moved to the UK at any time from the 1940s to the present day, or whose immediate family did so;
- to examine whether the experiences of health and wellbeing and healthcare access for these participants have been impacted by periods of uncertain residency or fragile citizenship.

Life storytelling methods (life story interviews) were utilised to achieve these aims, by producing short biographical accounts of these participants' lives and the lived experiences of health, wellbeing and healthcare access as Caribbean migrants.

Life story method for understanding health and wellbeing

A life story or life history story is an individual account about a person's life that can cover the time from birth to the present and can be presented in a variety of forms (Atkinson, 2007). It is a useful tool for examining migration journeys, because it generates insights into the social fields that are of importance in situations of mobility (Fog Olwig, 1999). It is also a technique that provides an opportunity to access and listen to the voices of marginalised and seldom heard groups, who are less visible and unheard in health research and healthcare systems. It can assist in addressing misconceptions about BME groups as being hard to reach, because it aims to give them 'the opportunity to tell his or her own story' and thus allows us to learn from their voice, their words and subjective meaning of their experience of life' and health (Atkinson, 2007: 233). By categorising BME groups as hard to reach in healthcare and health research, we can come to perceive BME people as a homogeneous group. This method, with the focus on the unique individual's experience, serves to prevent this from occurring. Life histories can therefore be used to increase our understanding of how people *individually* experience and adapt to major life events.

Life stories or life history stories have not been utilised extensively in healthcare research. However, they have been utilised in sociological research for some time, and are most famously known in the early work of the Chicago School at the start of the 20th century (Roberts, 2001; Harrison, 2008). Life stories or life histories were referred to by Chicago sociologists as written stories, but also included diaries, personal documents and secondary sources that could give an insight into the history of the individual (Roberts, 2001). This method was perceived by Chicago sociologists as being important for understanding the individual's feelings, perceptions, conceptions but also the interrelation between the individual and their social context (Harrison, 2008).

Since this period, the life story method has been approached by varying sociological perspectives. The epistemological, ontological and theoretical approaches adopted can impact on the type of methodological approach and analytical framework utilised (Clough et al, 2004). It is important to look briefly at the meaning of epistemology, ontology and common approaches that inform life history research.

Broadly, and in its simplest form, 'epistemology' refers to the study of knowledge (the forms of knowledge) and how we reach it. It is commonly understood as 'how we know what we know'; our ways of knowing and learning about social reality (Crotty, 1998: 8). The epistemology adopted will impact on the entire research process. There are various epistemological approaches towards life stories, and the central branches are either positivist or interpretivist. *Positivist* approaches focus on a scientific outlook on knowledge and will look at the data collected via life stories objectively. Positivist life story research therefore is more commonly quantitative. Quantitative methods are utilised to check on the accuracy and reliability of the personal histories and narratives and the validity of interpretations (Roberts, 2001). In contrast, *interpretivist* approaches towards life stories perceive knowledge and data as never being fully objective and as being removed from the research process. Interpretivists are interested in specific, contextualised environments and acknowledge that reality and knowledge are not objective but influenced by people within that environment. This approach focuses on subjective experience, and recognises that data is subject to biases, thus cannot be generalised in the way that positivist research can be.

'Ontology' refers to what constitutes reality and the researcher's stance towards the nature of knowledge. The ontological position will also impact on the way in which the life stories are delivered, understood and analysed. Ontological approaches refer to either objectivism (realist) or constructionism. A realist paradigm focuses on the belief in an objective form or reality and there is an empirical basis for individual experiences. Realists claim that there is an external reality, independent of what people may think or understand it to be. In contrast, a constructivist paradigm focuses on the construction of reality and its prominence in life stories. This approach maintains that reality can only be understood via the human mind and socially constructed meanings. Put more simply, individuals create subjective meanings of their experience and the world that are negotiated within the social, cultural and historical context in which their lives are embedded (Crotty, 1998).

The various theoretical approaches that are adopted and informed by the epistemological or ontological position of the researcher include, for example, ethnomethodology, phenomenology, narrative analysis, and symbolic interactionism. For further discussion of these approaches, see Roberts (2001) and Harrison (2008).

The theoretical approach adopted in this research is symbolic interactionism, informed by an interpretivist epistemological position and a constructivist stance to reality and the nature of knowledge. Therefore, the life histories allow for an interest in the specific and contextualised environments of the Caribbean migrants and that the realities and knowledge produced via this method are influenced by the people within that environment. From the constructivist position, it allows for a focus on how people construct the reality of their lives in their life stories. The symbolic interactionist approach adopted for this research is embedded in the principles of constructivism; thus, allowing for understanding of how individuals construct their identities and knowledge through interaction (Mead, 1934; Blumer, 1969).

This approach is useful for examining the experiences of health, health inequalities and healthcare access for BME groups, because it draws attention to power in racism and discrimination. Specifically, it allows for examination of the role that society and its interactions can play in generating and maintaining marginalised identities and inequalities.

As discussed in Chapter 2, constructivist approaches are commonly used to help us understand how shared meanings of race and ethnicity, and the marginalisation that accompanies them, are constructed in the history, traditions, practices and language of people (Du Bois, 1968; Chandra, 2001; Eriksen, 2002; Chandra and Wilkinson, 2008; Johnson et al, 2019).

Life story interviews: data collection

Life story data collection tools take a variety of forms and are applied differently across various disciplines. They are either autobiographical accounts, written by the individual, or biological accounts, in which the narrative is elicited via interviews or other formats completed by a researcher or biographer. They can be examined via personal documents and diaries, blogs, letters, autobiographical accounts/ journals and photographs and artwork (Harrison, 2008). Interviews are commonly used either independently or in combination with other personal narrative sources.

In this research, life story interviews were utilised, in which the researcher interviewed participants. The data collection tools used for life story interviews are either structured, semi-structured or unstructured. The question or questions presented can be selective or unselective. The approach adopted here included the selective and semi-structured life story interview, adapted from that approach developed by McAdams (1988). The interview guide was divided into several sections that asked the participant to discuss their life story since moving to the UK and identify a few key scenes in their life. Specifically, they were asked to describe the most important things that have happened in their life; that could include the happiest or saddest moments. They were also asked to think about their life as a book or novel, in which they develop a chapter title and describe briefly what each chapter is about.

Next, the participant was asked to identify key points, scenes or periods in their life story that included a *health* problem, challenge or crisis, and discuss in further depth. Probes were given here to understand their experiences with the NHS as a Caribbean migrant at that time. Additionally, participants were asked to comment on their overall health prior to moving to the UK and at the time of the interview, particularly with reference to the current COVID-19 pandemic and lockdown restrictions that were in place at the time of writing the research.

These scenes or periods are understood within McAdams's approach as critical life episodes – types of event or specific life experiences that took place at a particular time and place in the person's life and which stand out for a particular reason (McAdams, 1988). The participant is also asked why this particular scene is important or significant in their life. There is an option in McAdams' (1988) framework to include questions about the future. In this research, the participant was asked instead whether their health had changed since living in the Caribbean, and probes were given to understand how they perceived their future health and healthcare access as Caribbean migrants. The aim here was to understand whether the migrants felt that their health, wellbeing and healthcare access had suffered as a result of their move to the UK and migrant status. See Table 7.1 for details of the interview guide.

Table 7.1: Life story interview guide

Topics to cover

Introduction

This is a life story interview in which I would like you to share your experiences of being a Caribbean migrant in the UK. The story is selective; it does not need to include everything that has ever happened to you. Instead, I will ask you to focus on a few key things, such as your experiences of health, wellbeing and healthcare access since your arrival to the UK and any periods of fragile citizenship that you and your family have had that may have impacted on this.

Life story

Everyone has a life story. I'm interested in key parts of your story. Please tell me about your life story since moving from the Caribbean, in about 5–10 mins or so if you can. Begin wherever you like and include whatever you wish.

What have been important moments in your life?

Probe: Please tell me about the happiest and saddest periods in your life.

If you had an opportunity to write the story of your life in a book what would the chapters be about?

So, please give each chapter a title, and tell me just a little bit about what each chapter is about. You can have as many chapters as you want within your story, but can I suggest between two and seven.

Probe: last chapter.

Now that you have described the overall outline of your life, I would like you to identify and describe a scene or period in your life, including the present time, wherein you or a close family member confronted a health problem, challenge or crisis.

Probe: Please describe in detail what the health problem is or was and how it developed. Please discuss any experience you had with the healthcare system regarding this crisis or problem and your experiences as a Caribbean migrant. Maybe think about what impact this has had on you and your overall life story.

Self

How would you describe yourself before you moved to the UK from the Caribbean? How would you describe your health at that time?

How would you describe your health now? Probe: has COVID-19 had any impact on this.

Do you think your health has changed over the years? How? Probe: healthcare access.

After reading the participant information sheet and the informed consent form, ten participants consented and were recruited via a snowball sample, ranging in age from 40 to 75 years. Due to the occurrence of the COVID-19 pandemic and imposed social contact restrictions, the participants were not interviewed face to face as planned, but rather over the telephone for one–two hours. The interviews were completed by the author, a mixed Black African-white British female, born in the UK, who has family members from the Caribbean. The participants self-identified their ethnicity as Black African-Caribbean, some of whom considered themselves as British and others who considered themselves as Caribbean. All had moved or migrated to the UK from the Caribbean between the 1950s and the 1990s. Participants had either travelled to the UK alone as young children, with or without their parents, or as young adults for the purposes of joining family or for employment, education and training, and to support Britain's employment infrastructure. They all had close or extended family members who had either migrated from the 1940s or were identified as being of the Windrush generation. Participants were either currently working in public sector roles – notably within health and social care, the civil service and manual occupations – or had retired from their role. While the majority had been impacted by what they understood as fragile citizenship or uncertain residency, none at the time had had their right to remain denied or faced deportation.

Transcription and analysis

On completion of the life story interviews, they were transcribed verbatim and interpreted via a thematic content analysis. To maintain anonymity, certain details of the participants, such as names and ages, have been changed. The focus of the thematic content analysis has been guided by the specific research aims and the life story interview guide topics. The interviews were analysed using a thematic approach modelled loosely around that adopted by others utilising life story methods to understand health (Cox et al, 2013).

The thematic analysis entailed an iterative process of critical thinking, questioning and categorising the content of the stories into codes about the experiences of the participants and their health. The stories were then re-read, and the codes were categorised in themes and compiled under a heading informed by the participants' own words. Each theme was then analysed for frequency and common characteristics.

A final list of primary themes was then developed, that focused on the health and wellbeing of African-Caribbean migrants and the links to their migratory experiences. These themes included: "I was healthier back home", trauma of the migrant experience, unequal access to healthcare and treatment, "COVID-19 are just echoes of the past for us" and "hope and the need for change".

Findings and discussion

Health and wellbeing: "I was healthier back home!"

When participants were asked about their health, a key theme emerged within their life stories. This theme, "I was healthier back home", concerned migrants' perceptions of their health in the UK and how this compared to their health when they lived "back home" in the Caribbean. When asked to describe their life stories, all of the participants began with memories of their former lives in the Caribbean, in which they felt they were much "happier" and "healthier". They all felt that since moving from the Caribbean, their health and wellbeing had deteriorated, and that the journey to the UK and experiences of living here had been detrimental to their health. They perceived 'good health' as being free from long-term (chronic health) conditions that included diabetes, hypertension, limited mobility and obesity. They also felt that 'good mental health' or 'wellbeing' involved being free of anxiety, and stress that included "no fears or worries" and being "carefree". For example:

> 'When I was home as a child, I was carefree, although at the time you probably didn't realise it ... I guess it's because we hadn't yet experienced the difficult life here. But looking back on it, you were just free ... they were some of the happiest and healthiest days of my life.' (African-Caribbean female, retired, early 60s)

> 'I had a relatively stable and happy life in the Caribbean. One that you can look back on and say, there was no real urgency or pressure, you could live carefree and not worry in the same way we have to hear.' (African-Caribbean male, retired, early 60s)

> 'I would definitely say my childhood was a very happy time, being back home in the Caribbean. I am a child born from my Windrush parents. My sister and I, and my older sister were born abroad, and we came over with my uncle. My health and just my mental self were better back home, ... but

it all changed here.' (African-Caribbean female, employed healthcare, mid-50s)

Despite the impact of ageing on their health deterioration (for all age groups), none of the participants considered themselves, at the time, to be in 'good health'. They attributed this to the migrant experiences that had shaped their lives. Limited access to healthier natural organic food sources, limited access to stress- and risk-free working environments, and limited access to culturally competent healthcare were perceived as the root causes of their poor health. Additionally, structural racism – that included social and economic disadvantage and racial discrimination in employment – also impacted on their health and that of their family members (Gee and Ford, 2011; Bailey et al, 2017). In the following extracts, three participants discuss the social and economic disadvantages they experienced as Caribbean migrant public sector employees, and how their health has not been considered or supported by their employers:

'I was in perfect health when I was back home, yes, I was younger, and doing lots more activities but here [in the UK] life takes a toll. It's not easy because you have to work harder for it and even then, you're still treated differently by employers.' (African-Caribbean male, manual public sector worker, retired, early 70s)

'I think my health here is worse ... it's just my obesity now ... because I do night shifts, I have no time to exercise and then I'm just sleeping. It's really hard with work and the children to find five minutes to exercise - it just doesn't happen. We also don't have access to better food like fruits ... It's also more relaxing in Trinidad, less stressful, fewer bills, and much shorter working hours.' (African-Caribbean female, healthcare keyworker, early 40s)

'When we came, our health wasn't a subject that anybody wanted to discuss here or was interested in. Everybody (employers) just told you to get on and work. You knew, if you went off sick, you would lose the pay and so we Caribbean people couldn't do that – it just wasn't available for us unlike white people on different contracts. And that's why I think so many of us have gotten sick. As we got older things became chronic, even though you might have had some serious health symptoms ... we just carried on working regardless. Nobody (employers) seemed interested in *our* health. You were there to work, not to be off stick. So, if you weren't feeling well, and were Caribbean you just got up and got to work, basically ... you couldn't say "I'm feeling tired" [laugh] so you just kept going on, until you really couldn't do it anymore. And that's where I think a number of my health issues have come from.' (African-Caribbean female, social care keyworker, retired, mid-60s)

These narratives are similar to those presented in Wray and Bartholomew's (2006) research, in which they examined the influence of migration on the health of older African-Caribbean people in the UK. They, too, found that Caribbean migrants experienced socioeconomic disadvantages, notably in experiences of employment, working longer hours, and insecure contracts with lower pay. Furthermore, migrants attributed these factors to their poor health. These inequalities in employment can potentially help to explain why higher rates of chronic health conditions among UK Caribbean migrants differ with those left behind at home in Caribbean countries (Lacey et al, 2019).

All of the participants in this research also felt that the healthcare here was significantly different to that offered in the home countries. The majority felt that their health was better understood by clinicians at home. Specifically, all felt that the Caribbean healthcare service, while economically limited, offered access to doctors and healthcare professionals who understood them, notably their differentiated experiences of health, and their accent or dialect:

'The healthcare system is different here. When you move to a new country, you figure out things are different and difficult for us here. The healthcare system is not good ... because in Trinidad the doctors understood you – but here they just don't hear and they don't listen to you.' (African-Caribbean female, retired, early 40s)

'The doctors here and especially the white doctors don't really understand what we Caribbean people are saying, they often don't listen properly ... so you don't want to ask questions because it becomes pointless.' (African-Caribbean female, public sector worker, retired, early 60s)

'I've found the healthcare system much easier to access than my Dad – but that's because I have the clinical knowledge and I ask questions or ask to get a second opinion. However, this hasn't been the same for my Dad, who is from the Windrush. One of the things that I found with that is that he had developed health problems because he hadn't been taking medication. The doctors didn't explain the medication to him properly and he didn't understand that he should have been taking one of the tablets – so he didn't take it, so of course this then led to problems that he shouldn't of have had. The repeat prescriptions for the medication didn't arrive and he got sick. Unless I went with him, they … the doctors didn't take the time to understand him and this is happening to a lot of Caribbean people … you know the elders who came earlier.' (African-Caribbean female, public sector worker, retired, mid-60s)

Relationship between health and wellbeing and migratory experiences of trauma

When asked about their migration journeys and health, four key themes emerged in the participants' life stories. The first of these concerns the migratory experiences of trauma, for example their journey to the UK and the treatment they received on arrival and during their post-migration experiences.

These experiences of "unseen trauma" included periods of isolation, uncertain residency and feelings of being unwanted. For many, these experiences were detrimental to their health and wellbeing or that of immediate family members. Previous research examining Caribbean migration has found that migrants have experienced a traumatic introduction to British society that encompasses feelings of alienation discomfort, marginalisation and a longing for being back home with family (Fog Olwig, 1999; Byron and Condon, 2008). Similarly, the life stories in this sample were replete with these narratives of trauma. These experiences were due to racism, and often entailed being treated as "unwanted", and "uncertain … fragile" residents or citizens.

As discussed earlier, research has shown that BME groups often experience marginalisation and racism within public institutions, leading to feelings of not belonging or of being an unwanted outsider or insecure citizen (Sutherland, 2006; Griffiths, 2021). Experiences of racism and indifferent treatment by white professionals can hint at tension and discord, and signal to feelings of not being welcome or accepted as British citizens. For many in this research, this meant that they felt continually marked as "outsiders" or "others" to white British citizens, who could still be subject to UK immigration controls through error and on exceptional grounds.

Although all of the participants had accessed British citizenship at the time of the interviews, they did not experience a belief in a common British identity that they presumed to be shared with other white British citizens. For the majority, these experiences of trauma resulted in self-identification as failed and insecure citizens or unwanted migrants. In order to be perceived as 'good' citizens, they continued to construct themselves as self-sufficient and emotionally resilient, but recognised the significant impact that this had on their mental health. The following are examples of the trauma that three participants experienced on their arrival and early journeys to the UK and how they responded in development of self-sufficiency and resilience. They also draw attention to the lack of mental health support and provision they received during these experiences. All of the participants travelled to the UK as children through family migration:

'I came to the UK with my sister, my grandma and my cousin. I think I was about six. It was such a big and horrific change because nobody [from the Caribbean] really got much help. One minute you're on the boat, then when you got here … you've not got people around you, like you had back home. And, you know you just had to get on with it. I think that's one of the biggest problems with our generation who came – there was no mental health support for the trauma of it all, the big, huge change. And, you know, just fitting in. Yeah, it was tough because you knew you weren't really wanted here. You didn't always feel happy. You were always concerned, but it was just a matter of being tough and saying to yourself "well you're here now, you're gonna to have get on with it" and be resilient to how people treat you.' (African-Caribbean female, social care worker, retired, mid-60s)

'In terms of mental wellbeing, I do think that our generation have had to deal with a lot of the unseen trauma; the disruption that we experienced and happiness we were all denied in early childhood, you know the relationship forming with others and dealing with different kind of racist situations we found ourselves in. So, I really feel that this is something that has gone on unseen and will never ever be talked about by authorities or dealt with either. We the Windrush generation ... the wave of people who came in the 60s, were definitely never offered any kind of support with the trauma of the journey and our experiences of just being unwanted. Our health wasn't a subject that anybody [authorities and health professionals] want to discuss too or were interested in. We did just learn to develop ... a lot of resilience.' (African-Caribbean female, civil servant, retired, late 60s)

'I came to England, in the early 60s, as a child. I came on my own on a flight, my Mum, my Aunt and her two sisters were already living in London. In those days, children, travelled on their own and the airhostess just looked after them. But at the beginning, it was awful here ... a lonely dark and dreary place because it was just my mom and my Aunt, and I didn't really know anybody or fit in at all. Back home, you were accustomed to having friends and families around you and then I got here, and it was cold ... it was dark, and you were told to "go back to where you came from". You just thought "what am I doing here". As I got older, I sort of a got used to being in this cold place. And tried to not let it bother me anymore and face up to the fact that I'm never going to be able to go back, my mum just couldn't get the money. You know you don't want to just feel sad all the time and lonely, so you had to get stronger ... emotionally, and deal with the difficult people here and just not fitting in. And maybe that's why, even now, I am comfortable being on my own ... I just got used to it.' (African-Caribbean female, health worker, retired, late 60s)

For many of the participants, the trauma of the migrant journey was also situated in the context of their interaction with immigration and in their applications for a British passport. Although all of the participants had attained the right to remain in the UK at the time of the interviews, some experienced trauma in immigration processes prior to accessing their citizenship. For example, in the following comments, two of the participants discuss the problems they encountered and the treatment they received when travelling:

'I came to the country when I was 10 years old. My parents were living in London, at the time. My father met me at

Southampton docks, because I came on a boat. I spent 10 days on the boat. My Auntie brought me because I couldn't have a passport in my own right, so I came on that passport. I experienced difficulty with my passport when I was 19. I applied for my own passport, but it kept getting rejected – it got rejected four times, apparently because my parents were unmarried. In the end, I was advised to go to a solicitor and pay to change my name to prove that I was the child of my parents, but it still got rejected. It eventually got accepted but only when I wanted a visa to go to America – I had to prove I had a job and provide details of savings, when I did this, I got my passport.' (African-Caribbean female, former public sector worker, retired, early 70s)

'Unlike family members and friends of mine, I processed, my rights to remain without any major difficulties, but I think this is because I came later in my twenties and I came on my own passport – not a parent's passport or anything. It was supposed to be British passport which said "citizen of the United Kingdom and colonies". However, on arrival and when travelling you were not always made to feel like you were a British citizen. Immigration officers were always quick to ask, "what is the purpose of your visit" and I remember them saying, "you're a not a real British citizen". Even though you're holding a passport, you don't expect to be questioned all the time about your right to enter the country, you were constantly made to feel unwanted. But you just accepted it and become resistant to it, it seemed to be in my opinion to be the normal thing for immigration officers to do to Caribbean people.' (African-Caribbean male, former service industry public sector worker, retired, early 60s)

As discussed earlier, migrants from the Caribbean who came to the UK from the 1940s onwards for the purposes of employment have described traumatic experiences while working (Wray and Bartholomew, 2006). These experiences are often entrenched in structural racism, as the majority of Caribbean migrants who came in the 1940s to 1960s were funnelled into low-grade posts with lowest pay and, as a consequence, faced economic disadvantages in other sectors of society. Many also believed they never had a real chance to be successful, no matter how hard they worked (Wray and Bartholomew, 2006; Watson, 2013; Goodfellow, 2019).

Similar experiences were identified among the participants' life stories and in their discussion of their parents' working lives. The trauma in the migrant journey included inequalities in employment and housing. As we saw earlier, the consequences for their personal health were significant, as the opportunities to look after one's health or to recognise the signs or risks for serious health conditions were neglected, often ignored and seen as not being a concern. Despite attaining access to citizenship, migrants still perceived themselves as being welcome only temporarily, as long as they committed to working hard and to being resilient. Many commented on the impact of structural racism on their health – not only for themselves, but also for their parents – as they experienced economic inequalities and disadvantage, which often kept them from enjoying an equal space in public life, and faced systematic disadvantage (Gee and Ford, 2011; Bailey et al, 2017). Specifically, the low pay and nature of work contracts, and the subsequent inequalities in accessing affordable and secure housing, meant that they, or older parents, were unable to stop working because of illness or to reduce working hours. For some, this resulted in, or contributed to, serious health conditions, but it also led to fatalities of older parents or relatives. For example, two of the female participants explained the impact that these inequalities had had on the health of their 'Windrush mothers' and their utilisation of healthcare:

> 'My mother was a Windrush migrant … we lost her to cancer when she was in her 60s. She didn't get the same entitlement to employment or rights regarding her health or welfare that other white British people got at that time. I remember it was terrible in those days especially when my mother got terminally ill, my father had to take on extra shifts because she could no longer work. But my mum just kept working for as long as she physically could and opted not to have treatment in order to keep … food on the table. She actually chose not to have lengthy and what was gruelling chemo treatment at that time, so she could keep working and receive an income. She felt that she had responsibilities to us kids, but it came to a point where she couldn't do that anymore and she just had to be up in her bed.' (African-Caribbean female, healthcare keyworker, mid-50s)

'My mom was one of the Windrush people who came in the 50s. She used to work in the health service. And, unbeknownst to us, apparently one day she must have been bad at work because they brought her home, but she didn't explain any of this to us. She hid her illness so she could continue to work. The next day, she went back to work. But she collapsed and one of her colleagues, came to the house and told us, that we need to take her to the doctor because she had a stroke or a heart attack. Although she was sick, she kept working because at that time we were having the problem with the house; ... we were being asked to leave, so she needed to keep working to keep it and she suffered for it, ... she eventually died in that house.'
(African–Caribbean female, retired, late 60s)

Although migration has led to a more ethnically diverse workforce in the NHS, several researchers have reported negative experiences of racism, marginalisation and discrimination for Black and Caribbean nurses that are similar to those presented in this research (Batnitzky and McDowell, 2011; Likupe and Archibong, 2013; Sands et al, 2020). Specifically, Sands et al (2020) found that Caribbean migrant nurses have been encouraged to accept lower positions that have fewer entitlements and rights than those offered to British white nurses. Female participants in this research who worked in the NHS services as nurses or healthcare professionals, also experienced similar experiences in their employment. Although all the women had been working in the NHS for some time (20–30 years), they all discussed the impact of discrimination and the ongoing impact this had to their health. For example, in the following extracts, three of the women describe the racism and discrimination they received:

'I thought that being in the caring NHS profession, if you were to become ill, somebody somewhere, would look after you the way you looked after the white British patients. But it's not what it seems. It's supposed to be a caring profession but not for me as a Caribbean nurse. They don't care about you as a person, you're just a number. No one has an interest in your health. If you become injured, or you're ill, they don't do the same, like what we do for the patients. And it's supposed to be a caring profession, but they certainly did not do that. You were told to train and work and be a caring professional, but you don't feel that they were caring in return. Once you got in, you just worked and serve the people who are here.' (African-Caribbean female, retired, late 60s)

'It never existed, there was no compassion shown towards us by the bosses, unlike what they did for white British nurses. But don't get me wrong, if we did our job well, then we got paid but because you are Caribbean, or a black person, you'd be treated differently, different shifts, different access to holiday time and in my case very different treatment when you got sick. I got seriously injured by a patient and have been housebound ever since. I was treated differently to the white British nurses who had similar experiences. They didn't go through what I went through. They got easier access to support, treatment and compensation for their injuries. They weren't told that they are "young tough and resilient" and that they'll be able to go back to work. As soon as they got injured, they were signed off work for good, but I was told to keep going and it took years before they were prepared to do something and even then, I was still treated differently.' (African-Caribbean female, retired, late 60s)

'As far as I'm concerned, there is institutional racism in the NHS and there still is. I experienced it in training and in trying to access my higher qualifications. Also, the fact is, even when you get there and get your qualifications, it takes you three times longer because you know you are different to others. When I was working white patients would never come to me, even though I was qualified to treat them, they would go to or ask for my white colleagues, and my colleagues would thrive on this. My bosses never recognised or treated me the same as the white less qualified staff.' (African-Caribbean female, mid 50s)

It has been suggested that Black Caribbean nurses face this racism and discrimination because they are perceived by employers and colleagues as not being British, and therefore not safe until accredited against British standards (Smith and Mackintosh, 2007). However, the narratives of the women presented in this research show that despite attaining accreditation and working in the NHS for over 20 years, the discrimination and marginalisation continued for them and consequentially impacted negatively on their physical and mental health.

What also appears to be significant here, is that there is a lack of regard and support within the NHS service provision for the overall health of the Caribbean employees from overseas. While measures such as the Equality Act 2010 and the Workplace Race Equality Charter may exist to prevent discrimination and to provide support for the health of BME NHS staff, these participants feel that access to services to support their health is inequitable. As one of the previous participants explained: "the NHS is a caring profession ... but just not for me".

A second significant theme articulated by all the participants concerned the relationship between inequalities in accessing healthcare and the impact on their health. All of the participants discussed negative interactions with the health service and its professionals. These either occurred for them directly or for family members, including parents, children and partners. The experiences spanned their life histories and occurred repeatedly for some. As discussed earlier, healthcare professionals 'back home' in the Caribbean were perceived by some to be more understanding of them (for example language) and their health "better". Common occurrences included racism by healthcare professionals in the form of racial stereotyping and marginalisation in access to treatment. Marginalisation focused on "being ignored" and "not listened" to by healthcare professionals, when presenting for diagnosis or treatment. This regularly resulted in medical conditions being missed or delayed in diagnosis. For example, one of the female participants explains her first experience of marginalisation within the healthcare system:

> 'The first time I saw how the healthcare system fail people like us from the Caribbean is when my grandmother died of stomach cancer. She would go to the doctor and sort of keep telling him about it. But he would just keep treating her for indigestion for years, even though she kept telling him it was more serious. Then when she was really poorly and she went into the hospital, but by then it was too late. They couldn't do anything, and she just died. You kind of just accept it, but it's a real failure of the NHS.' (African-Caribbean female, retired health and social care worker, early 60s)

Racial stereotyping when being diagnosed or treated in healthcare was discussed by the participants as being common in their lives. Participants felt that many practitioners held assumptions about their bodies that focused on them possessing 'strong' and 'resilient working' black bodies that require limited physical health intervention. However, when their damaged or less functioning black bodies are presented for diagnosis or treatment, the cause of the medical condition is either ignored, or often attributed to the deviant behaviour of the Caribbean person.

Research in this area, supports these findings, and has shown that clinicians and medical students can hold false beliefs about the differences between black and white patients. This influences racial bias and stereotyping in pain perceptions and treatment recommendations (Hoffman et al, 2016). These forms of racial stereotyping in diagnosis and treatment were discussed by the participants. This is evidenced in the following comment made by two participants in their discussion of access to healthcare for themselves and their family members:

'My husband experienced racism during a consultation recently. He's quite fit, because he was an athlete back home … in field events. But when we came here, he started having these really bad hip pains. So, we saw the doctor and he sent him off for an X-ray and further tests. We then discovered that he had to have a total hip replacement. However, when the consultant was doing the examination, he had some of the medical students with him, and he asked them: "why do you think this relatively fit man has to have a total hip replacement at his age?" One of them responded and said, "it's because of the drugs he's taken over the years!". We laughed at the time, but we look back now and realise that is how we are always seen … you know … troublesome and that our health is our fault in some way.' (African–Caribbean female, healthcare worker, early 40s)

'I have not been given the opportunity to receive the best possible treatment that was available at the time. When, when you appear to be physically able, even when you're feeling ill, the opportunities to go for an X-ray, further treatment or a second stage of treatment are usually seen as not being an option. They assume you're fit and strong because you're from the Caribbean. The doctor doesn't always say okay, I'll send you for an X-ray. The doctor in his assessment will look at you from a physical point of view, and think you look really physically fit and say, "you may have just pulled a muscle". Yet, you will be suffering from an injury from working in the industry for all these years, but the doctor is reluctant to send you for that second opinion. And for that reason, you may not have received the best possible assessment of your circumstances. We've been working all these years just pushing through the pain but when you just can't cope with the medical situation with which you're faced the doctors aren't very support. Also, Caribbean people are not good complainers. They don't really complain. And so very often, doctors don't very often give you time and Caribbean people very often suffer from not getting the best possible service from the health service.' (African-Caribbean male, former service industry public sector worker, retired, early 60s)

The belief that Caribbean people, notably older generations, don't complain about their health was discussed by all of the participants and recognised as being common. While this implies that Caribbean migrant elders are making themselves hard to reach to healthcare professionals, what should be considered is the historical and social context that may have contributed to and informed this behaviour. Historical experiences of racism and discrimination in healthcare access and ongoing economic and social disadvantage across society, have led to a tradition of self-reliance, self-sufficiency and minimising of health issues among Caribbean elder migrants (Bailey and Tribe, 2021).

In this research, participants revealed that this tradition has been informed by their Caribbean parents and relatives who arrived earlier in the UK from the 1940s, but this has been transferred across and down through generations. However, the participants also felt that Caribbean people have continued to receive negative experiences within the NHS, that has inhibited future help-seeking, created a self-sufficient outlook and led to a reluctance among some to discuss health difficulties or to question health professionals (Truswell, 2019; Bailey and Tribe, 2021). These practices become embedded in practice and help to explain help-seeking among some Caribbean people. To improve misconceptions of these BME groups as being hard to reach and inaccessible in healthcare services we therefore need to examine both historical and recent experiences of racism and discrimination in healthcare access and public institutions that impact on health-seeking practice.

When asked about their health and COVID-19, a third theme emerged that concerned "echoes of the past". All the participants commented on the high number of deaths of COVID-19 among BME groups that had recently been reported in public media. All felt that social and economic disadvantages experienced by BME people who had died from COVID-19, was "no different" to what they or their parents had experienced on arriving to the UK and living in the UK as a Caribbean migrant. For them, "nothing has changed". Specifically, the structural racism that included inequalities in employment were echoes of their past, and had just highlighted the ongoing causal factors that already existed for BME people. Furthermore, treatment of current Black Caribbean staff within the NHS – that included low-paid and high-risk roles, limited access to PPE and long shifts – were indicators of their social and economic disadvantages and the unequal treatment they were accustomed to while working. For example, this is discussed by three of the participants, who had previously worked, or were currently working, as NHS nurses:

'COVID right now and being locked in is no different for me because I've been in lockdown since 1992. I was injured by a patient. I've been treated the same as the NHS BME staff on the front line now … it's just echoes of the past for us [Caribbean people] nothing has changed. It's actually getting worse because I've spoken to Caribbean nurses who are still working and nothing has changed, it's still the same experiences for us. You would have thought by now [since the Windrush], that they'd start to look after the staff, but they don't care. I feel with Covid-19, more Caribbean nurses and staff, are obviously dying from COVID because they do all the donkey work. You see similar treatment or even exactly the same treatment now; look at who's working on the COVID wards, all the black nurses and yet, we are the ones getting injured and dying. So, to me, nothing has changed.' (African-Caribbean female, retired healthcare worker, early 60s)

'I'm working on a COVID ward now because I got moved from my ward to help. It's a really scary experience working on the ward, because you are worrying all the time about coming home. I don't want to bring it to my family, you see it in the media about the black and ethnic minority staff getting it and dying. A couple of black colleagues have had it really bad and our bosses were constantly ringing them to see when they can come back in. You look at the statistics in the hospitals and you're just thinking "oh my god what if I bring it home to my husband, will he be able to survive?" So, it's always going through my mind … it's tough for me. Also, the government say they are risk assessing black and ethnic minority staff, but not one person to this day have come to any of us. Also, one of my other black colleagues, caught it at work and her whole family was tested positive for COVID. The manager was calling her and asking, "when are you coming back out to work" and she had to go back in. That's the thing it's just delivery, rather than care for people like us. It feels like nothing has changed from the past.' (African-Caribbean female, healthcare worker, early 40s)

'I feel like they treat me differently, I've been asking for the risk assessment because I'm BME staff but I'm still waiting. One minute they tell me I'm high risk and yet I've not had the assessment. I've been chasing for weeks and weeks now … I'm fed up of trying, I've given up. I've just got to keep working … I don't have a choice. But it's no different to how it's always been for people like us.' (African-Caribbean female, healthcare worker, mid 40s)

A fourth and final theme voiced by all of the participants, was the idea of "hope" and the "need for change" in access to equitable healthcare. All of the participants recognised the need for change in the access to healthcare and the right to remain in the UK, but importantly wanted to see a decline in structural racism and discrimination for people like themselves who had moved from the Caribbean. None of the participants in the study had personally had their right to remain in the UK denied at the time of the interviews, and all were classified as British citizens. However, the majority discussed the negative impact of their migration journeys and its impact on their health, all of which were embedded in experiences of racism, discrimination and marginalisation in healthcare access and wider sectors of society. Those who had fewer personal experiences of these inequalities witnessed them for their older family members.

It is these migrant experiences that informed their narratives of hope and the need for change to the health of Caribbean people and their healthcare access. Specifically, they wanted much further recognition and support to be given to those who had been mentally and physically impacted by Caribbean migration. They also wanted reparation for the racism and marginalisation experienced in employment and various sectors of society that accompanied this fragile identity. For example, one female participant explained:

'I think the whole experience you know … moving here as a child, the work and the healthcare has had a bigger impact on your mental health that people are aware of. More needs to be done to change this. The impact to your physical health has also been tough. I've been unwell since my 30s, and it's a bit of a life sentence with the medication. I think my blood pressure has been impacted by the whole ongoing experience … I only hope they do more and change it for us.' (African-Caribbean female, retired health and social care worker, early 60s)

In addition to the provision of mental health provision and support, some of the participants wanted public apologies and adequate compensation to be given to those who had sustained the racism and economic disadvantages and were working in high-risk public sector roles. They also recognised the role that intersectionality played in their health inequalities. Specifically, they acknowledged how migrants with fewer skills, limited education and low incomes faced greater disadvantages in accessing healthcare and citizenship. Therefore, they hoped for change in addressing this and supporting those Caribbean people who experience multiple discriminations. This is evidenced in the comments made by two of the participants:

'The government, employers and healthcare should apologise to the people that came from every part of the Caribbean to help and support public services. It hasn't been fair to some people who couldn't read or write properly and now can't stay. But also, to the people like us who have been treated badly … for the racism and different access.' (African-Caribbean male, former public sector worker, retired, early 70s)

'I can't say I have really felt it *as much* as others in healthcare who have been treated differently or not got access because of their passports, but it still needs to change for other people I know who were not as educated and knowledgeable as me and haven't be able to stay. As I said I got rejected numerous times … but I could pay for a solicitor numerous times.' (African-Caribbean female, former service industry public sector worker, retired, early 60s)

Conclusion

This chapter has provided a brief insight in to how a group of African-Caribbean heritage have experienced their health, wellbeing and healthcare access since arriving in the UK. The participants in this research have arrived at different times since the 1940s until the 1990s. Many were children of what they described as "Windrush parents", who arrived in the 1940s. Others arrived later, from the 1970s, for the purposes of work and to be with family who had previously migrated.

While many were not impacted directly by the hostile environment policy in which they have faced deportation, all provide a telling insight into their difficult migrant journeys and experiences. For the majority of these participants, their migrant identities involved fragility or uncertainty, and these are attributed to experiences of trauma, discrimination and inequality that have existed across their lives but also in the lives of their family members. These experiences have impacted their physical health and mental wellbeing and those of their immediate family members.

None of the participants perceived themselves as being in good health. They all reported existing chronic health conditions that included diabetes, hypertension, cancer, mobility issues, disability and obesity. They also felt that "good mental health" or "wellbeing" involved being free of anxiety and stress that included "no fears or worries" and being "carefree". They all felt that since moving from the Caribbean, their health and wellbeing had deteriorated, and that the journey to the UK and experiences of living here had been detrimental to the health. This led them to perceive "their health as being better back at home in the Caribbean".

Reasons for their poor health have been attributed to limited access to: healthier, natural organic food sources; stress-free and risk-free working environments; and culturally competent healthcare. Additionally, structural racism (that included social and economic disadvantage) and racial discrimination in employment, immigration and wider public institutions were also influential. These were identified as periods of trauma, including feelings of being unwanted and experiences of working longer hours, in high-risk roles, on insecure contracts with lower pay. These were experienced not only by the participants themselves, but also by their elders, who arrived in the 1940s.

Experiences of inequality and discrimination were also identified in their access to healthcare and treatment. Notably, experiences of racial bias and stereotyping in diagnosis and treatment led them to perceive the NHS and its professionals as lacking cultural competency. NHS professionals and service providers were perceived as having a lack of understanding of Caribbean people – their differentiated health conditions, medication requirements, dialect and health-seeking behaviour. It was also recognised that help-seeking among some Caribbean people is embedded in historical experiences of racism and discrimination in healthcare access and public institutions that can lead to self-sufficient behaviour and an unwillingness to express health concerns. This can lead to misconceptions of these groups as being hard to reach by healthcare professionals.

However, the historical discriminations of Caribbean migrants in public institutions and the ongoing experiences of racism have led to a mistrust in public institutions and in the NHS. In order to move beyond this misconception, the theme that focused on echoes of the past is important. It draws attention to the inequalities in health and healthcare access for BME groups, and the factors influencing this have not changed. Marginalisation and racism in its various forms have been, and continue to be, influential.

But what does this mean for our research and healthcare practices? The narratives of hope and change identified by the participants can help to inform guidance to address marginalisation and racism for us as practitioners and researchers. Urgent calls for mental health and wellbeing programmes to address the post-traumatic impact of the hostile environment on the Windrush generation and their descendants are needed (Vernon, 2019), but they should *also* be provided to Caribbean people who have migrated and been able to access healthcare. This is because they still face inequalities, discrimination and marginalisation that have significantly impacted on their mental and physical health.

Also, the role of intersectionality in ethnic health inequalities must also be considered. We can no longer assume that our research and healthcare practices or provision can be applied homogeneously to understand and address the health inequalities experienced by African-Caribbean migrants or any other BME group. The life story methods employed here have provided an insight into the individual and differentiated migrant journeys that are impacted by multiple discriminations. Specifically, education, employment type, income and age all impact on the disadvantages that Caribbean migrants experience in accessing healthcare and fragile and certain citizenship.

Life story methods are a useful research tool that can help to achieve this, but providing individual accounts that are inherently missing in Home Office, health service and health research enquiries or evaluations, but also contextualise these with an exploration of wider economic, social and political factors. They can also provide insights into long-term change (social, economic, political) that may have occurred in addressing ethnic health inequalities. But, as we have seen here, there doesn't seem to be much change. Rather, the association between ethnicity, race and COVID-19 incidence is just an indicator on the ongoing wider determinants of health that have impacted – and continue to impact – on BME people.

Recommendations for health researchers and practitioners are to employ alternative or additional methods, such as life history methods or stories, in order to understand Caribbean migration and its impact on health, health inequalities and healthcare access. However, in order to identify these migrants in healthcare settings and beyond, researchers need to do much more to identify the migration status of African-Caribbean groups and other BME groups. As discussed, there is an inherent lack of inclusion and standardisation in the conceptualisation and categorisation of migration status in health research and routine administrative health systems. This highly complicates our access to health information and understanding of migration experiences (Bhopal, 2014). Life story methods can assist to capture this, but practitioners and researchers must take more action to provide research evidence that captures health outcomes by migration status (for example country of birth, duration of residence, nature of migration status) for African-Caribbean groups in the UK (Bhopal, 2014). As we have seen, mortality data (for example death registration) in the UK relies predominantly on country of birth, incidence and prevalence data by ethnicity, which makes it difficult to understand patterns for non-communicable health conditions among migrants (Jayaweera, 2014).

Conclusion

Throughout this book, it has been argued that we need to think differently about the terms we employ when doing inclusive practice in health and health-related research. In this book, the terms 'BME' and 'ethnic minority groups' have referred to any other ethnic grouping apart from white British. The terms and typologies we use to identify and classify people from different ethnic backgrounds and racial groups impact on how these groups are understood and interpreted by others. Importantly, we need to avoid use of the term 'hard to reach', because it problematises BME and ethnic minority groups and assumes that they are solely responsible for their health and healthcare access.

As we have seen, terms such as this can be utilised by dominant and majority groups to legitimise hierarchies and to maintain segregation, marginalisation and discrimination towards minorities. Recognition of this is important, because research in this field, and presented here, acknowledges that people from different ethnic backgrounds and racial groups are still being treated differently by health service providers and feel unequal to White British groups (Salway et al, 2016; Race Disparity Unit, 2019a). Furthermore, perceived discrimination among minority groups is relatively high in healthcare settings and can lead to them forgoing healthcare (Rivenbark and Ichou, 2020).

The research presented in this book – and specifically in Chapters 5, 6 and 7 – has shown that BME groups are not hard to reach, but rather we need to do more to improve the way in which we design and deliver services for them and complete research with or about them. Specifically, we need to improve the methods and practices we utilise to understand their health and healthcare access and the factors that impact on these.

This book has also shown that there is a paucity of national public health resources that examine health inequalities and its causes. There are also significant problems in the recording and monitoring of ethnicity and its classifications, which contributes to an invisibility of ethnic minority groups in health research and public health data. Notably, in Chapter 1 it was demonstrated that the meaning of race and ethnicity is often misunderstood and conflated, and there are diverse variations in the concepts used to define ethnic minorities. BME group categories are also often applied homogeneously and generalised across diverse groups. Furthermore, it was evidenced in Chapter 3 that the recording and monitoring of ethnicity and/or race in health research is often missed, ignored or collected incorrectly. This results in exclusionary practices, in which BME groups are presumed to be less visible in health research, and the various intersecting wider determinants of health are misunderstood or not explored in depth.

The research presented here, in Chapters 5, 6 and 7, has paid closer attention to the multiple and additional intersecting dimensions of BME identities that impact on their marginality and differentiated experiences of health and healthcare access. Additional dimensions of intersectionality, such as religion and/or faith, migration status, and location, are important for understanding how BME groups in this research experienced their health and accessed health interventions (Reimer-Kirkham and Sharma, 2011; Mwangi and Constance-Huggins, 2017; Collins and Bilge, 2020).

In light of these findings, we – as researchers and practitioners – need to work more with these presumed to be hard-to-reach groups, to understand how intersectionality is relevant for their health, health inequalities and access to healthcare. As has been evidenced, there are minimal studies in the UK that facilitate a focus on this approach and its impact on health and access to healthcare interventions for BME people (Tomalin et al, 2019). However, it is evident from the research presented here that these groups are not necessarily hard to reach for the delivery of health and lifestyle behaviour change programmes, but rather they are perceived as invisible and therefore the programmes do not reach them. Consequently, to address their perceived invisibility, an intersectional lens is required for creating programmes, and this should be applied in our evaluation of such provision. However, application of this approach cannot be standardised and homogeneous, in which we assume these dimensions of marginality are relevant for all people within an ethnic group; rather, we need to understand what other dimensions exist for them and how they apply specifically to the groups and/or individuals involved.

This book has wider implications for health research policy, healthcare practice and the methods used in health research and healthcare to examine ethnic health. It is evident that there are legal duty requirements for public healthcare services to demonstrate equal treatment across all areas of delivery and access to healthcare (Equality Act 2010). However, there is limited inclusion for improving the equality practice of researchers and the evaluation of its impact on health research and health monitoring.

As health research informs the commissioning of future healthcare provision, research funding councils and bodies should devise further policies to ensure that funded research focuses on improving the equality practices of researchers. There should be equality training that is informed and designed collaboratively with BME groups. Furthermore, there should be mandatory equality monitoring, cultural competency training and equality impact assessments that provide more than online 'tick box' training packages for staff and researchers.

This book also has implications for the methods we use to understand health, health inequalities and healthcare access for BME groups. Here it has been shown that we need to improve the recording and monitoring of ethnicity and race in health research and healthcare practice. While the incentives to improve ethnicity coding under the Quality and Outcomes Framework have helped to improve monitoring, the training mentioned earlier should be provided and should include much further guidance on the differences between race and ethnicity.

It should also illustrate the importance of collecting ethnicity and data, and how to record ethnicity competently. The methods we use should also consider the inclusion of qualitative approaches, such as life story methods and open space techniques, where possible (McAdams, 1988; Atkinson, 1998, 2007, Harrison, 2008). However, where this is less feasible in clinical and evaluative trials, we should continue to improve our equality practices and consider how health and physical activity screening tools, such as the IPAQ (Cora et al, 2003), can be culturally adapted in collaboration with BME groups to improve our equality practices.

The implications of this book for healthcare practice are that cultural sensitivity should be considered further in the commissioning, design and evaluation of healthcare and health and lifestyle interventions. While culturally sensitive approaches do exist, there must be further recognition of the trauma, fragility of identity and discrimination experienced by BME groups. As this research has shown, BME groups still face inequalities, discrimination and marginalisation in their healthcare and access to wider society, which have significantly impacted on their mental and physical health.

In light of this, we need to be more cautious about the practices we utilise in both healthcare and research practice that can exacerbate perceptions of discrimination and distrust among ethnic minority groups. The lack of inclusionary practice can potentially increase health disparities among these groups and encourage them to become hard to reach.

Hopefully this book has provided some basic guidance for researchers and practitioners on how to avoid misconceptions of BME groups as being hard to reach – and how to deliver services and research that may help to understand their experiences of health and healthcare access. By improving practice, we can introduce change and give greater meaning to the statement that 'black lives matter ... and should not be forgotten in healthcare and research' (Matt Hancock, UK Secretary of State for Health and Social Care, House of Lords, 3 June 2020).

References

Abdalla, S., Cronin, F., Daly, L., Drummond, A., Fitzpatrick, P., Frazier, K., Hamid, N., Kelleher, C., Kelly, C., Kilroe, J., Lotya, J., McGorrian, C., Moore, R.G., Murnane, S., Nic Charthaigh, R., O'Mahony, D., O'Shea, B., Quirke, B., Staines, A., Staines, D., Sweeney, M.R., Turner, J., Ward, A. and Whelan, J. (2010) *All Ireland Traveller Health Study – Our geels: Summary of findings*. University College Dublin. Available at: https://health.gov.ie/wpcontent/uploads/2014/03/AITHS2010_SUMMARY_LR_All.pdf, accessed 20/08/2020.

Adkison-Bradley, C., Maynard, D., Johnson, P. and Carter, S. (2009) British African-Caribbean women and depression. *British Journal of Guidance & Counselling*, 37(1), pp.65–72.

Agyemang, C., Bhopal, R. and Bruijnzeels, M. (2005) Negro, Black, Black African, African Caribbean, African American or what? Labelling African origin populations in the health arena in the 21st century. *Journal of Epidemiology of Community Health*, 59, pp.1014–1018.

Agyemang, C., Humphry, R.W. and Bhopal, R. (2012) Divergence with age in blood pressure in African-Caribbean and white populations in England: Implications for screening for hypertension. *American Journal of Hypertension*, 25(1), pp.89–96.

Agurs-Collins, T.D., Kumanyika, S.K., Ten Have, T.R. and Adams-Campbell, L.L. (1997) A randomized controlled trial of weight reduction and exercise for diabetes management in older African American subjects. *Diabetes Care*, 20(10), pp.1503–1511.

Allik, M., Brown, D., Dundas, R. and Leyland, A.H. (2019) Differences in ill health and in socioeconomic inequalities in health by ethnic groups: A cross-sectional study using 2011 Scottish census. *Ethnicity & Health*, 17 July, pp.1–19.

Ambikaipaker, M. (2018) *Political Blackness in Multiracial Britain*. Philadelphia: University of Pennsylvania Press.

Anand, A.S. and Cochrane, R. (2005) The mental health status of South Asian women in Britain: A review of the UK literature. *Psychology and Developing Societies*, 17(2), pp.195–214.

Andrews, K. (2016) The problem of political blackness: Lessons from the Black Supplementary School Movement. *Ethnic and Racial Studies*, 39(11), pp.2060–2078.

Arai, L. and Harding, S. (2004) A review of the epidemiological literature on the health of UK-born Black Caribbeans. *Critical Public Health*, 14(2), pp.81–116.

Arnott, P. (2019) *Windrush: A ship through time*. Stroud: The History Press.

Arredondo, E.M., Mendelson, T., Holub, C., Espinoza, N. and Marshall, S. (2012) Cultural adaptation of physical activity self-report instruments. *Journal of Physical Activity & Health*, 9(Suppl 1), pp.S37–S43.

Arthur, C.A.R. and Rowe, A.A. (2012) Black women and diabetes, in L. Jack Jr. (ed.) *Diabetes in Black America: Clinical and public health solutions to a national crisis*. Chicago: Hilton Publishing, pp.187–217.

Aspinall, P.J. (2003) Who is Asian? A category that remains contested in population and health research. *Journal of Public Health Medicine*, 25(2), pp.91–97.

Aspinall, P.J. (2011) The utility and validity for public health of ethnicity categorization in the 1991, 2001 and 2011 British Censuses. *Public Health*, 125 (10), pp.680–687.

Atkinson, R. (1998) *The Life Story Interview*. Thousand Oaks, CA: Sage.

Atkinson, R. (2007) The life story interview as a bridge in narrative inquiry, in D.J. Clandinin (ed.) *Handbook of Narrative Inquiry: Mapping a methodology*. London: Sage, pp.224–245.

Atkinson, R. and Flint, J. (2001) Accessing hidden and hard-to-reach populations: Snowball research strategies. *Social Research Update*, 33(1), pp.1–4.

Babakus, W.S. and Thompson, J.L. (2012) Physical activity among South Asian women: A systematic, mixed-methods review. *International Journal of Behavioral Nutrition and Physical Activity*, 9(1), pp.9–150.

Bailey, N.V. and Tribe, R. (2021) A qualitative study to explore the help-seeking views relating to depression among older Black Caribbean adults living in the UK. *International Review of Psychiatry*, 33(1–2), pp.113–118.

Bailey, Z.D., Krieger, N., Agénor, M., Graves, J., Linos, N. and Bassett, M.T. (2017) Structural racism and health inequities in the USA: Evidence and interventions. *The Lancet*, 389(10077), pp.1453–1463.

Bamidele, O.O., E. McGarvey, H., Lagan, B.M., Chinegwundoh, F., Ali, N. and McCaughan, E. (2019) 'Hard to reach, but not out of reach': Barriers and facilitators to recruiting Black African and Black Caribbean men with prostate cancer and their partners into qualitative research. *European Journal of Cancer Care*, 28(2), p.e12977.

Barkan, E. (1992) *The Retreat of Scientific Racism: Changing concepts of race in Britain and the United States between the World Wars*. Cambridge: Cambridge University Press.

Barnett, K., Mercer, S.W., Norbury, M., Watt, G., Wyke, S. and Guthrie, B. (2012) Epidemiology of multimorbidity and implications for health care, research, and medical education: A cross-sectional study. *Lancet*, 380(9836), pp.37–43.

Batnitzky, A. and McDowell, L. (2011) Migration, nursing, institutional discrimination and emotional/affective labour: Ethnicity and labour stratification in the UK National Health Service. *Social Cultural Geography*, 12(2), pp.181–201.

Bauer, G.R. (2014) Incorporating intersectionality theory into population health research methodology: Challenges and the potential to advance health equity. *Social Science and Medicine*, 110, pp.10–17.

Bayar, M. (2009) Reconsidering primordialism: An alternative approach to the study of ethnicity. *Ethnic and Racial Studies*, 32(9), pp.1639–1657.

BBC (2018) May apologises to Caribbean leaders, 17 April. *UK Politics*. Available at: https://www.bbc.com/news/uk-politics-43792411, accessed 27/07/2020.

Becker, E., Boreham, R., Chaudhury, M., Craig, R., Deverill, C., Doyle, M., Erens, B., Falaschetti, E., Fuller, E. and Hills, A. (2006) *Health Survey for England 2004: The health of minority ethnic groups*. London: National Centre for Social Research.

Beder, H.W. (1980) Reaching the hard-to-reach adult through effective marketing. *New Directions for Continuing Education*, 8, pp.11–26.

Bell, S., Clarke, R., Mounier-Jack, S., Walker, J.L. and Paterson, P. (2020) Parents' and guardians' views on the acceptability of a future COVID-19 vaccine: A multi-methods study in England. *Vaccine*, 38(49), pp.7789–7798.

Bennett, N.R., Francis, D.K., Ferguson, T.S., Hennis, A.J., Wilks, R.J., Harris, E.N., MacLeish, M.M. and Sullivan, L.W. (2015) Disparities in diabetes mellitus among Caribbean populations: A scoping review. *International Journal for Equity in Health*, 14(1), p.23.

Benoit, C., Jansson, M., Millar, A. and Phillips, R. (2005) Community-academic research on hard-to-reach populations: Benefits and challenges. *Qualitative Health Research*, 15(2), pp.263–282.

Berthoud, R. and Bryan, M. (2011) Income, deprivation and poverty: A longitudinal analysis. *Journal of Social Policy*, 40(1), pp.135–156.

Bhavnani, R., Mirza, H.S. and Meetoo, V. (2005) *Tackling the Roots of Racism: Lessons for success*. Bristol: Policy Press.

Bhopal, R.S. (1997) Is research into ethnicity and health racist, unsound, or important science? *BMJ*, 314(7096), pp.1751–1756.

Bhopal, R.S. (2007) *Ethnicity, Race, and Health in Multicultural Societies: Foundations for better epidemiology, public health, and health care.* Oxford: Oxford University Press.

Bhopal, R.S. (2014) *Migration, Ethnicity, Race, and Health in Multicultural Societies.* Oxford: Oxford University Press.

Bhopal, R.S. (2019) *Epidemic of Cardiovascular Disease and Diabetes: Explaining the phenomenon in South Asians worldwide.* Oxford: Oxford University Press.

Bhopal, R.S. (2020) Delaying part of PHE's report on covid-19 and ethnic minorities turned a potential triumph into a PR disaster. *BMJ Opinion.* Available at: https://blogs.bmj.com/bmj/2020/06/16/delaying-part-of-phes-report-on-covid-19-and-ethnic-minorities-turned-a-potential-triumph-turned-into-a-pr-disaster/, accessed 06/07/2020.

Bhopal, R. and Donaldson, L. (1998) White, European, Western, Caucasian, or what? Inappropriate labelling in research on race, ethnicity, and health. *American Journal of Public Health*, 88(9), pp.1303–1307.

Bhopal, R. and Rankin, J. (1999) Concepts and terminology in ethnicity, race and health: Be aware of the ongoing debate. *British Dental Journal*, 186(10), pp.483–484.

Bilge, S. (2009) Smuggling intersectionality into the study of masculinity: Some methodological challenges. *Feminist Research Methods: An international conference, University of Stockholm* (Vol. 4, No. 9, February).

Blumer, H. (1969) *Symbolic Interactionism: Perspective and method.* Berkeley: University of California Press.

Bonilla-Silva, E. (1996) Rethinking racism: Toward a structural interpretation. *American Sociological Review*, 62(3), pp.465–480.

Bopp, M., Wilcox, S., Hooker, S.P., Butler, K., McClorin, L., Laken, M., Saunders, R. and Parra-Medina, D. (2007) Peer reviewed: Using the RE-AIM Framework to evaluate a physical activity intervention in churches. *Preventing Chronic Disease*, 4(4), A87.

Bostock, N. and Haynes, L. (2020) COVID-19 death rate highest among BAME groups, delayed PHE review confirms. *GPOnline.com.* Available at: https://www.gponline.com/covid-19-death-rate-highest-among-bame-groups-delayed-phe-review-confirms/article/1684962, accessed 02/06/2020.

Bowleg, L. (2012) The problem with the phrase women and minorities: Intersectionality—an important theoretical framework for public health. *American Journal of Public Health*, 102(7), pp.1267–1273.

Bowleg, L., Teti, M., Malebranche, D.J. and Tschann, J.M. (2013) 'It's an uphill battle everyday': Intersectionality, low-income Black heterosexual men, and implications for HIV prevention research and interventions. *Psychology of Men & Masculinity*, 14(1), pp.25–34.

Brangan, E., Stone, T.J., Chappell, A., Harrison, V. and Horwood, J. (2019) Patient experiences of telephone outreach to enhance uptake of NHS Health Checks in more deprived communities and minority ethnic groups: A qualitative interview study. *Health Expectations*, 22(3), pp.364–372.

Brathwaite, A.C. and Lemonde, M. (2017) Exploring health beliefs and practices of Caribbean immigrants in Ontario to prevent Type 2 diabetes. *Journal of Transcultural Nursing*, 28(1), pp.15–23.

Breach, A. and Yaojun, L. (2017) *Gender Pay Gap by Ethnicity in Britain – Briefing*. The Fawcett Society, March. Available at: https://www.fawcettsociety.org.uk/Handlers/Download.ashx?IDMF=f31d6adc-9e0e-4bfe-a3df-3e85605ee4a9, accessed 14/09/2018.

Brink, H., Van der Walt, C. and Van Rensburg, G. (2006) *Fundamentals of Research Methodology for Health Care Professionals*. Cape Town: Juta and Company Ltd.

British Heart Foundation (2001) *Coronary Heart Disease Statistics. Diabetes Supplement*. London: BHF.

British Heart Foundation (2010) *Ethnic Differences in Cardiovascular Disease*. Oxford: BHF.

Broca, P. (1864) *On the Phenomena of Hybridity in the Genus Homo*. London: for the Anthropological Society, by Longman, Green, Longman, & Roberts.

Brown, K., Avis, M. and Hubbard, M. (2007) Health beliefs of African–Caribbean people with Type 2 diabetes: A qualitative study. *British Journal of General Practice*, 57(539), pp.461–469.

Butler, C., Tull, E.S., Chambers, E.C. and Taylor, J. (2002) Internalized racism, body fat distribution, and abnormal fasting glucose among African-Caribbean women in Dominica, West Indies. *Journal of the National Medical Association*, 94(3), p.143.

Byron, M. and Condon, S. (2008) *Migration in Comparative Perspective: Caribbean communities in Britain and France* (Vol. 6). London: Routledge.

Cabinet Office (2019a) *Ethnicity Facts and Figures, Common Mental Disorder*. Available at: https://www.ethnicity-facts-figures.service.gov.uk/health/mental-health/adults-experiencing-common-mental-disorders/latest#full-page-history, accessed 23/06/2020.

Cabinet Office (2019b) *Tackling Inequalities Faced by Gypsy, Roma and Traveller Communities, Seventh Report of Session 2017–19*. Women and Equalities Committee, House of Commons. Available at: https://publications.parliament.uk/pa/cm201719/cmselect/cmwomeq/360/full-report.html#heading-8, accessed 04/07/2020.

Caiola, C., Docherty, S., Relf, M. and Barroso, J. (2014) Using an intersectional approach to study the impact of social determinants of health for African-American mothers living with HIV. *Advances in Nursing Science*, 37(4), pp.287–298.

Candler, T.P., Mahmoud, O., Lynn, R.M., Majbar, A.A., Barrett, T.G. and Shield, J.P.H. (2018) Continuing rise of Type 2 diabetes incidence in children and young people in the UK. *Diabetic Medicine*, 35(6), pp.737–744.

Caperchione, C.M., Kolt, G.S. and Mummery, W.K. (2009) Physical activity in culturally and linguistically diverse migrant groups to Western society. *Sports Medicine*, 39(3), pp.167–177.

Carbado, D.W., Crenshaw, K.W., Mays, V.M. and Tomlinson, B. (2013) Intersectionality: Mapping the movements of a theory. *Du Bois Review: Social Science Research on Race*, 10(2), pp.303–312.

Chakraborty, A.P.U. and McKenzie, K. (2002) Does racial discrimination cause mental illness? *British Journal of Psychiatry*, 180(6), pp.475–477.

Chamberlain, M. (2003) Rethinking Caribbean families: Extending the links. *Community, Work & Family*, 6(1), pp.63–76.

Chandra, K. (2001) Introduction. *APSA-CP: Newsletter of the Organized Section in Comparative Politics of the American Political Science Association*, 12(1), pp.7–11.

Chandra, K. and Wilkinson, S. (2008) Measuring the effect of 'ethnicity'. *Comparative Political Studies*, 41(4–5), pp.515–563.

Chang, V.W., Hillier, A.E. and Mehta, N.K. (2009) Neighborhood racial isolation, disorder and obesity. *Social Forces: A Scientific Medium of Social Study and Interpretation*, 87(4), pp.2063–2092.

Chaturvedi, N. (2003) Ethnic differences in cardiovascular diseases. *Heart*, 89, pp.681–686.

Chouhan, K. and Nazroo, J. (2020) Health inequalities, in B. Byrne, C. Alexander, O. Khan, J. Nazroo and W. Shankley (eds) *Ethnicity, Race and Inequality in the UK, State of the Nation*. Bristol: Bristol University Press, pp.73–92.

Clough, P., Goodley, D., Lawthom, R. and Moore, M. (2004) *Researching Life Stories: Method, theory and analyses in a biographical age*. London: Routledge.

Cole, E.R. (2009) Intersectionality and research in psychology. *American Psychologist*, 64(3), pp.170–180. Available at: http://dx.doi.org/10.1037/a0014564, accessed 13/09/2018.

Cole, M. (2020) *Theresa May, the Hostile Environment and Public Pedagogies of Hate and Threat: The case for a future without borders.* London: Routledge.

Collins, P.H. (1990) *Black Feminist Thought: Knowledge, consciousness, and the politics of empowerment.* New York: Routledge.

Collins, P.H. and Bilge, S. (2016) *Intersectionality.* Malden, MA: Polity Press.

Collins, P.H. and Bilge, S. (2020) *Intersectionality.* Cambridge: Polity Press.

Comstock, R.D., Castillo, E.M. and Lindsay, S.P. (2004) Four-year review of the use of race and ethnicity in epidemiologic and public health research. *American Journal of Epidemiology*, 159(6), pp.611–619.

Condon, L., Bedford, H., Ireland, L., Kerr, S., Mytton, J., Richardson, Z. and Jackson, C. (2019) Engaging gypsy, Roma, and Traveller communities in research: Maximizing opportunities and overcoming challenges. *Qualitative Health Research*, 29(9), pp.1324–1333.

Cook, D. (2002) Consultation, for a change? Engaging users and communities in the policy process. *Social Policy & Administration*, 36(5), pp.516–531.

Cooper, C., Morgan, C., Byrne, M. and Dazzan, P. (2008) Perceptions of disadvantage, ethnicity and psychosis. *British Journal of Psychiatry*, 192, pp.185–190.

Cooper, R. and David, R. (1986) The biological concept of race and its application to public health and epidemiology. *Journal of Health Politics, Policy and Law*, 11, pp.97–116.

Cora, C., Marshall, A.L., Sjostrom, M., Bauman, A.E., Booth, M.L., Ainsworth, B.E., Pratt., M., Ulf, E., Agneta, Y., James, S. and Oja, P. (2003) International Physical Activity Questionnaire: 12-country reliability and validity. *Medicine and Science Sports and Exercise*, 35(8), pp.1381–1395.

Cox, K.S., Casablanca, A.M. and McAdams, D.P. (2013) 'There is nothing good about this work': Identity and unhappiness among Nicaraguan female sex workers. *Journal of Happiness Studies*, 14(5), pp.1459–1478.

Craig, G. and Atkin, K. (eds) (2012) *Understanding 'Race' and Ethnicity: Theory, history, policy, practice.* Bristol: Policy Press.

Crenshaw, K. (1989) Demarginalizing the intersection of race and sex: A Black feminist critique of antidiscrimination doctrine, feminist theory, and antiracist politics. *University of Chicago Legal Forum*, 139(1), pp.139–167.

Crenshaw, K. (1991) Mapping the margins: Intersectionality, identity politics, and violence against women of color. *Stanford Law Review*, 43, pp.1241–1299.

Creswell, J.W. and Poth, C.N. (2017) *Qualitative Inquiry and Research Design: Choosing among five approaches.* London: Sage.

Cromarty, H. (2019) *House of Commons Library: Briefing Paper Number 08083: 9 May: Gypsies and Travellers.* Briefing paper, House of Commons Library.

Crotty, M. (1998) *The Foundations of Social Research: Meaning and perspective in the research process.* London: Sage.

Crowe, S., Cresswell, K., Robertson, A., Huby, G., Avery, A. and Sheikh, A. (2011) The case study approach. *BMC Medical Research Methodology*, 11(1), p.100.

Darwin, C. (1859) *The Origin of the Species.* London: J. Murray.

De Maynard, V.A. (2007) An ethnographic study of Black men within an inner London area to elicit relatedness between Black human condition and the onset of severe mental illness: What about the Black human condition? *International Journal of Mental Health*, 36(4), pp.26–45.

Dennis, R.M. (1995) Social Darwinism, scientific racism, and the metaphysics of race. *The Journal of Negro Education*, 64(3), pp.243–252.

Department of Health (2001) *National Service Framework for Diabetes.* Available at: www.dh.gov.uk/en/Publicationsandstatistics/Publications/PublicationsPolicyAndGuidance/Browsable/ DH_4096591, accessed 20/08/2020.

Department of Health (2002) *Addressing Inequalities: Reaching the hard-to-reach groups.* National Service Frameworks. Available at: https://webarchive.nationalarchives.gov.uk/20120503231542/http://www.dh.gov.uk/en/Publicationsandstatistics/Publications/PublicationsPolicyAndGuidance/DH_4005259, accessed 29/05/2020.

Diabetes UK (2010) *Diabetes in the UK 2010 Key Statistics on Diabetes.* Diabetes UK. Available at: https://www.diabetes.org.uk/resources-s3/2017-11/diabetes_in_the_uk_2010.pdf, accessed 24/08/2018.

Diabetes UK (2016) *Facts and Stats.* Available at: https://www.diabetes.org.uk/Documents/Position%20statements/DiabetesUK_Facts_Stats_Oct16.pdf, accessed 24/08/2018.

Diabetes UK (2018) *Facts and Figures.* Available at: https://www.diabetes.org.uk/professionals/position-statements-reports/statistics, accessed 24/10/2018.

Doherty, P., Stott, A. and Kinder, K. (2004) *Delivering Services to Hard to Reach Families in On Track Areas: Definition, consultation and needs assessment.* London Research, Development and Statistics Directorate: Home Office, pp.1–12.

Douglas, J. (2016) Developing an intersectionality based framework for health promotion, in *22nd International Union of Health Promotion and Education World Conference, 22–26 May 2016, Curitiba, Brazil.*

Douglas, J. (2018) The politics of Black women's health in the UK: Intersections of 'race,' class, and gender in policy, practice, and research, in J.S. Jordan-Zachery and N.G. Alexander-Floyd (eds) *Black Women in Politics: Demanding citizenship, challenging power, and seeking justice.* Albany: State University of New York Press, pp.49–68.

Du Bois, W.E.B. (1940) *Dusk of Dawn: An essay toward an autobiography of a race concept.* New Brunswick: Transaction Publishers.

Du Bois, W.E.B. (1968) *The Souls of Black Folk: Essays and sketches.* Chicago: A.G. McClurg, 1903. New York: Johnson Reprint Corp.

Edge, D. (2008) 'We don't see Black women here': An exploration of the absence of Black Caribbean women from clinical and epidemiological data on perinatal depression in the UK. *Midwifery*, 24(4), pp.379–389.

Edge, D. (2013) Why are you cast down, o my soul? Exploring intersections of ethnicity, gender, depression, spirituality and implications for Black British Caribbean women's mental health. *Critical Public Health*, 23(1), pp.39–48.

Edge, D., Degnan, A. and Rafiq, S. (2020) Researching African-Caribbean mental health in the UK: An assets-based approach to developing psychosocial interventions for schizophrenia and related psychoses, in R. Majors, K. Carberry and T. Ranshaw (eds) *The International Handbook of Black Community Mental Health.* Bingley: Emerald Publishing Limited, pp.455–470.

Edwards, R. and Holland, J. (2013) *What is Qualitative Interviewing?* London: Bloomsbury.

Ehtisham, S., Kirk, J., McEvilly, A., Shaw, N., Jones, S., Rose, S., Matyka, K., Lee, T., Britton, S.B. and Barrett, T. (2001) Prevalence of Type 2 diabetes in children in Birmingham. *BMJ*, 322, p.1428.

Ellard-Gray, A., Jeffrey, N.K., Choubak, M. and Crann, S.E. (2015) Finding the hidden participant: Solutions for recruiting hidden, hard-to-reach, and vulnerable populations. *International Journal of Qualitative Methods*, 14(5), https://doi.org/10.1177/1609406915621420.

El-Sayed, A.M., Scarborough, P. and Galea, S. (2011) Ethnic inequalities in obesity among children and adults in the UK: A systematic review of the literature. *Obesity Reviews*, 12(5), pp.e516–e534.

Eriksen, T.H. (2002) *Ethnicity and Nationalism: Anthropological perspectives, culture, anthropology and society series*, 2nd edn. London: Pluto Press.

Fanzana, B.M. and Srunv, E.A. (2001) A venue-based method for sampling hard-to-reach populations. *Public Health Reports*, 116(1), pp.216–222.

Farmaki, A.E., Garfield, V., Eastwood, S.V., Farmer, R.E., Mathur, R., Giannakopoulou, O.O., Patalay, P., Kuchenbaecker, K., Sattar, N., Hughes, A. and Bhaskaran, K. (2020) Type 2 diabetes risks and determinants in 2nd generation migrants and mixed ethnicity people of South Asian and African Caribbean descent in the UK. *medR*, xiv, pp.2019–12.

Fenton, S. (2003) *Ethnicity*. Cambridge: Polity Press.

Ferguson, L.D., Ntuk, U.E., Celis-Morales, C., Mackay, D.F., Pell, J.P., Gill, J.M.R. and Sattar, N. (2018) Men across a range of ethnicities have a higher prevalence of diabetes: Findings from a cross-sectional study of 500 000 UK Biobank participants. *Diabetic Medicine*, 35(2), pp.270–276.

Firdous, T., Darwin, Z. and Hassan, S.M. (2020) Muslim women's experiences of maternity services in the UK: Qualitative systematic review and thematic synthesis. *BMC Pregnancy and Childbirth*, 20(1), pp.1–10.

Fisher, K.A., Bloomstone, S.J., Walder, J., Crawford, S., Fouayzi, H. and Mazor, K.M. (2020) Attitudes toward a potential SARS-CoV-2 vaccine: A survey of U.S. adults. *Annals of Internal Medicine*, 173(12), 964–973.

Flanagan, S.M. and Hancock, B. (2010) 'Reaching the hard to reach': Lessons learned from the VCS (voluntary and community sector). A qualitative study. *BMC Health Services Research*, 10(1), https://doi.org/10.1186/1472-6963-10-92.

Fog Olwig, K. (1999) Narratives of the children left behind: Home and identity in globalised Caribbean families. *Journal of Ethnic and Migration Studies*, 25(2), pp.267–284.

Ford, C.L. and Airhihenbuwa, C.O. (2010) Critical race theory, race equity, and public health: Toward antiracism praxis. *American Journal of Public Health*, 100(S1), pp.S30-S35.

Forouhi, N.G., Merrick, D., Goyder, E., Ferguson, B.A., Abbas, J., Lachowycz, K. and Wild, S.H. (2006) Diabetes prevalence in England 2001: Estimates from an epidemiological model. *Diabetic Medicine*, 23(2), pp.189–197.

Freimuth, V.S. and Mettger, W. (1990) Is there a hard-to-reach audience? *Public Health Reports*, 105(3), pp.232–238.

Gabriel, R.H. (1940) *The Course of American Democratic Thought*. New York: Ronald Press.

Gaglio, B., Shoup, J.A. and Glasgow, R.E. (2013) The RE-AIM framework: A systematic review of use over time. *American Journal of Public Health*, 103(6), pp.e38–46.

Gagné, T. and Veenstra, G. (2017) Inequalities in hypertension and diabetes in Canada: Intersections between racial identity, gender, and income. *Ethnicity & Disease*, 27(4), pp.371–378.

Galton, F. (1883) *Inquiries into Human Faculty and its Development.* London: Macmillan & Co.

Gee, G.C. and Ford, C.L. (2011) Structural racism and health inequities: Old issues, new directions. *Du Bois Review: Social Science Research on Race*, 8(1), pp.115–132.

Gee, G., Ro, A., Shariff-Marco, S. and Chae, D. (2009) Racial discrimination and health among Asian Americans: Evidence, assessment, and directions for future research. *Epidemiologic Reviews*, 31(1), pp.130–151.

Gee, G.C., Walsemann, K.M. and Brondolo, E. (2012) A life course perspective on how racism may be related to health inequities. *American Journal of Public Health*, 102(5), pp.967–974.

Geertz, C. (1973) *The Interpretation of Cultures.* New York: Basic Books.

Gentleman, A. (2019) *The Windrush Betrayal: Exposing the hostile environment.* London: Faber & Faber.

George, J., Mathur, R., Shah, A.D., Pujades-Rodriguez, M., Denaxas, S., Smeeth, L., Timmis, A. and Hemingway, H. (2017) Ethnicity and the first diagnosis of a wide range of cardiovascular diseases: Associations in a linked electronic health record cohort of 1 million patients. *PloS One*, 12(6), e0178945. doi: 10.1371/journal.pone.0178945

Germain, S. and Yong, A. (2020) COVID-19 highlighting inequalities in access to healthcare in England: A case study of ethnic minority and migrant women. *Feminist Legal Studies*, 28, pp.301–310.

Giritli Nygren, K. and Olofsson, A. (2014) Intersectional approaches in health-risk research: A critical review. *Sociology Compass*, 8(9), pp.1112–1126.

Glasgow, R.E., Vogt, T.M. and Boles, S.M. (1999) Evaluating the public health impact of health promotion interventions: The RE-AIM framework. *American Journal of Public Health*, 89(9), pp.1322–1327.

Glennerster, R. and Hodson, N. (2020) Confused out of care: Unanticipated consequences of a 'hostile environment'. *Journal of Medical Ethics*, 46(3), pp.163–167.

Glover, G. and Evison, F. (2009) *Use of New Mental Health Services by Ethnic Minorities in England.* Durham, England: North East Public Health Observatory. Available at: http://www.nepho.org.uk/publications /782/, accessed 22/06/2020.

Goff, L.M. (2019) Ethnicity and Type 2 diabetes in the UK. *Diabetic Medicine*, 36(8), pp.927–938.

Goodfellow, M. (2019) *Hostile Environment: How immigrants became scapegoats*. London: Verso Books.

Gould, S. (1980) *The Panda's Thumb: More reflections in natural history*. New York: W.W. Norton & Company.

Gramlich, J. and Funk, C. (2020) *Black Americans Face Higher COVID-19 Risks, Are More Hesitant to Trust Medical Scientists, Get Vaccinated*. Pew Research Centre. Available at: https://www.pewresearch.org/fact-tank/2020/06/04/black-americans-face-higher-covid-19-risks-are-more-hesitant-to-trust-medical-scientists-get-vaccinated/, accessed 01/01/2020.

Grant, C. (2019) *Homecoming: Voices of the Windrush Generation*. London: Random House.

Green, J. and Thorogood, N. (2018) *Qualitative Methods for Health Research*. London: Sage.

Griffith, D.M., Metzl, J.M. and Gunter, K. (2011) Considering intersections of race and gender in interventions that address US men's health disparities. *Public Health*, 125(7), pp.417–423.

Griffiths, M. (2021) 'My passport is just my way out of here': Mixed-immigration status families, immigration enforcement and the citizenship implications. *Identities*, 28(1), pp.18–36.

Grills, C.N., Aird, E.G. and Rowe, D. (2016) Breathe, baby, breathe: Clearing the way for the emotional emancipation of Black people. *Critical Methodologies*, 16(3), pp.333–343.

Haines, L., Wan, K.C., Lynn, R., Barrett, T.G. and Shield, J.P.H. (2007) Rising incidence of Type 2 diabetes in children in the U.K. *Diabetes Care*, 30, pp.1097–1101.

Halkier, B. and Jensen, I. (2011) Doing 'healthier' food in everyday life? A qualitative study of how Pakistani Danes handle nutritional communication. *Critical Public Health*, 21(4), pp.471–483.

Halpern, D. and Nazroo, J. (2000) The ethnic density effect: Results from a national community survey of England and Wales. *International Journal of Social Psychiatry*, 46(1), pp.34–46.

Hammarström, A. and Hensing, G. (2018) How gender theories are used in contemporary public health research. *International Journal for Equity in Health*, 17(1), p.34. Available at: https://doi.org/10.1186/s12939-017-0712-, accessed 02/04/2021.

Hanif, W., Ali, S.N., Patel, K. and Khunti, K. (2020) Cultural competence in Covid-19 vaccine rollout. *BMJ*, 371, m4845. Available at: https://www.bmj.com/content/371/bmj.m4845/rr, accessed 04/12/2021.

Harrison, B. (ed.) (2008) *Life Story Research*. London: Sage.

Harrison, G., Owens, D., Holton, A., Neilson, D. and Boot, D. (1988) A prospective study of severe mental disorder in Afro-Caribbean patients. *Psychological Medicine*, 18(3), pp.643–657.

Hayes, L., White, M., Unwin, N., Bhopal, R., Fischbacher, C., Harland, J. and Alberti, K.G.M.M. (2002) Patterns of physical activity and relationship with risk markers for cardiovascular disease and diabetes in Indian, Pakistani, Bangladeshi and European adults in a UK population. *Journal of Public Health*, 24(3), pp.170–178.

Health Foundation (2020) *Health Equity in England: The Marmot Review 10 years on*. Institute of Health Equity. Available at: http://www.instituteofhealthequity.org/resources-reports/marmot-review-10-years-on/the-marmot-review-10-years-on-full-report.pdf, accessed 26/06/2020.

Health Survey for England (2017) *01 Jan 2017 to 31 Dec 2017, 4th Dec 2018*. Available at: https://digital.nhs.uk/data-and-information/publications/statistical/health-survey-for-england/2017, accessed 31/01/2019.

Heard, E., Fitzgerald, L., Wigginton, B. and Mutch, A. (2019a) Applying intersectionality theory in health promotion research and practice. *Health Promotion International*, 35(4), pp.866–876. Available at: https://academic.oup.com/heapro/article/doi/10.1093/heapro/daz080/5544760, accessed 08/07/2020.

Heard, E., Fitzgerald, L., Va'ai, S., Collins, F., Whittaker, M. and Mutch, A. (2019b) 'In the Islands people don't really talk about this stuff, so you go through life on your own': An arts-based study exploring intimate relationships with young people in Samoa. *Culture, Health & Sexuality*, 21(5), pp.526–542. Available at: https://www.tandfonline.com/doi/abs/10.1080/13691058.2018.1492021, accessed 08/07/2010.

Heim, D., Hunter, S.C. and Jones, R. (2011) Perceived discrimination, identification, social capital, and well-being: Relationships with physical health and psychological distress in a UK minority ethnic community sample. *Journal of Cross-Cultural Psychology*, 42(7), pp.1145–1164.

Henderson, J., Gao, H. and Redshaw, M. (2013) Experiencing maternity care: The care received and perceptions of women from different ethnic groups. *BMC Pregnancy Childbirth*, 13(196).

Hesse-Biber, S.N. and Leavy, P. (2010) *The Practice of Qualitative Research*. London: Sage.

Hex, N., Bartlett, C., Wright, D., Taylor, M. and Varley, D. (2012) Estimating the current and future costs of Type 1 and Type 2 diabetes in the UK, including direct health costs and indirect societal and productivity costs. *Diabetic Medicine*, 29(7), pp.855–862.

Higginbottom, G.M.A. (2006) African Caribbean hypertensive patients' perceptions and utilization of primary health care services. *Primary Health Care Research & Development*, 7(1), pp.27–38.

Higgins, V., Nazroo, J. and Brown, M. (2019) Pathways to ethnic differences in obesity: The role of migration, culture and socio-economic position in the UK. *SSM-Population Health*, 7. doi: 10.1016/j.ssmph.2019.100394

HM Government (2015) *Sporting Future: A new strategy for an active nation*. London: Sport England.

HMO Health and Safety Executive (2004) *Successful Interventions with Hard to Reach Groups*. Available at: http://www.hse.gov.uk/research/misc/hardtoreach.pdf, accessed 05/05/2020.

Hoffman, K.M., Trawalter, S., Axt, J.R. and Oliver, M.N. (2016) Racial bias in pain assessment and treatment recommendations, and false beliefs about biological differences between blacks and whites. *Proceedings of the National Academy of Sciences*, 113(16), pp.4296–4301.

Hogan, V.K., de Araujo, E.M., Caldwell, K.L., Gonzalez-Nahm, S.N. and Black, K.Z. (2018) 'We black women have to kill a lion everyday': An intersectional analysis of racism and social determinants of health in Brazil. *Social Science & Medicine*, 199, pp.96–105.

Hoppitt, T., Shah, S., Bradburn, P., Gill, P., Calvert, M., Pall, H., Stewart, M., Fazil, Q. and Sackley, C. (2012) Reaching the 'hard to reach': Strategies to recruit black and minority ethnic service users with rare long-term neurological conditions. *International Journal of Social Research Methodology*, 15(6), pp.485–495.

House of Lords (2020) *Covid-19 Response* (3 June 2020). Available at: https://hansard.parliament.uk/lords/2020-06-03/debates/D3160B41-7311-4F63-B6E1-D04076375736/Covid-19Response, accessed 27/08/2020.

Huang, Y.T., Ma, Y.T., Craig, S.L., Wong, D.F.K. and Forth, M.W. (2020) How intersectional are mental health interventions for sexual minority people? A systematic review. *LGBT Health*, 7(5), pp.220–236. Available at: https://doi.org/10.1089/lgbt.2019.0328, accessed 10/07/2020.

Husain, M.I., Waheed, W. and Husain, N. (2006) Self-harm in British South Asian women: Psychosocial correlates and strategies for prevention. *Annals of General Psychiatry*, 5(1). Available at: https://doi.org/10.1186/1744-859X-5-7, accessed 02/04/2021.

Husain, N., Cruickshank, K., Husain, M., Khan, S., Tomeson, B. and Rahman, A. (2012) Social stress and depression during pregnancy and in the postnatal period in British Pakistani mothers: A cohort study. *Journal of Affective Disorders*, 140(3), pp.268–276.

ICNARC (2020) *ICNARC report on COVID-19 in critical care 12 June 2020*. Available at: https://www.icnarc.org/Our-Audit/Audits/Cmp/Reports, accessed 12/06/2020.

Iqbal, G., Johnson, M.R., Szczepura, A., Gumber, A., Wilson, S. and Dunn, J.A. (2012) Ethnicity data collection in the UK: The healthcare professional's perspective. *Diversity and Equality in Health and Care*, 9(4), pp.281–290.

Jayaweera, H. (2014) *Health of Migrants in the UK: What do we know?* Briefing paper. Centre on Migration, Policy and Society. University of Oxford.

Jefferys, M. (2006) *Teaching Cultural Competence in Nursing and Health Care*. New York: Springer.

Jenson, A.R. (1869) How can we boost IQ and scholastic achievement. *Harvard Education Review*, 39, pp.1–123.

Johnson, J.L., Bottorff, J.L., Browne, A.J., Grewal, S., Hilton, B.A. and Clarke, H. (2004) Othering and being othered in the context of health care services. *Health Communication*, 16(2), pp.255–271.

Johnson, M.R.D., Bhopal, R.S., Ingleby, J.D., Gruer, L. and Petrova-Benedict, R.S. (2019) A glossary for the first World Congress on Migration, Ethnicity, Race and Health. *Public Health*, 172, pp.85–88.

Jomeen, J. and Redshaw, M. (2013) Ethnic minority women's experience of maternity services in England. *Ethnic Health*, 18(3), pp.280–296.

Jones, M. and Kai, J. (2007) Capturing ethnicity data in primary care: Challenges and feasibility in a diverse metropolitan population. *Diversity in Health and Social Care*, 4(3), pp.211–220.

Joseph Rowntree Foundation (2017) *Poverty and Ethnicity in the Labour Market*. Joseph Rowntree Foundation. Available at: https://www.housingnet.co.uk/pdf/Poverty_ethnicity_round_up_Sep17.pdf, accessed 25/06/2020.

Karasz, A., Dempsey, K. and Fallek, R. (2007) Cultural differences in the experience of everyday symptoms: A comparative study of South Asian and European American women. *Culture, Medicine and Psychiatry*, 31(4), pp.473–497.

Karasz, A., Gany, F., Escobar, J., Flores, C., Prasad, L., Inman, A., Kalasapudi, V., Kosi, R., Murthy, M., Leng, J. and Diwan, S. (2019) Mental health and stress among South Asians. *Journal of Immigrant and Minority Health*, 21(Suppl 1), pp.7–14.

Karlsen, S., Becares, L. and Roth, M. (2012) Understanding the influence of ethnicity and health, in G. Craig, K. Atkin, S. Chattoo and R. Flynn (eds) *Understanding 'Race' and Ethnicity: Theory, history, policy, practice*. Bristol: Policy Press, pp.115–32.

Karlsen, S., Nazroo, J.Y. and Smith, N.R. (2020) Ethnic, religious and gender differences in intragenerational economic mobility in England and Wales. *Sociology,* 54(5), pp.883–903. Available at: https://doi.org/10.1177/0038038520929562, accessed 06/07/2020.

Karlsen, S., Nazroo, J.Y., McKenzie, K., Bhui, K. and Weich, S. (2005) Racism, psychosis and common mental disorder among ethnic minority groups in England. *Psychological Medicine,* 35(12), pp.1795–1803.

Keating, F. (2007) *African and African Caribbean men and mental health. Better Health Briefing Paper 5.* Available at: http://www.raceeequalityfoundaiton. org.uk/, accessed 22/06/2020.

Keating, F. (2019) *Socially-oriented Approaches to Recovery for African and Caribbean Men,* Research Findings 83. London: NIHR School for Social Care Research.

Keating, F. and Robertson, D. (2004) Fear, black people and mental illness: A vicious circle. *Health and Social Care in the Community,* 12(5), pp.439–447.

Kelly, M. and Nazroo, J.Y. (2018) Ethnicity and health, in G. Scambler (ed.) *Sociology as Applied to Medicine.* 7th edn. Oxford: Elsevier, pp.159–175.

Khan, O. (2012) *A Sense of Place: Retirement decisions among older Black and minority ethnic people.* London: Runnymede Trust. Available at: https://www.runnymedetrust.org/uploads/publications/pdfs/ASenseOfPlace-2012.pdf, accessed 13/09/2018.

Khanam, S. and Costarelli, V. (2008) Attitudes towards health and exercise of overweight women. *The Journal of the Royal Society for the Promotion of Health,* 128(1), pp.26–30.

Khunti, K., Morris, D.H., Weston, C.L., Gray, L.J., Webb, D. and Davies, M.J. (2013) Joint prevalence of diabetes, impaired glucose regulation, cardiovascular disease risk and chronic kidney disease in South Asians and White Europeans. *PLoS One,* 8(1), e55580.

Kid, B. (1902) *Principles of Western Civilisation.* New York: Macmillan.

Knight, M., Bunch, K., Tuffnell, D., Jayakody, H., Shakespeare, J., Kotnis, R., Kenyon, S. and Kurinczuk, J.J. (2018) *MBRRACE-UK, Saving Lives, Improving Mothers' Care.* Available at: https://www.npeu.ox.ac.uk/downloads/files/mbrrace-uk/reports/MBRRACE-UK%20Maternal%20Report%202018%20-%20Web%20Version.pdf, accessed 03/07/2020.

Knight, M., Bunch, K., Kenyon, S., Tuffnell, D. and Kurinczuk, J.J. (2020a) A national population-based cohort study to investigate inequalities in maternal mortality in the United Kingdom, 2009–17. *Paediatric and Perinatal Epidemiology,* 34(4), pp.392–398.

Knight, M., Bunch, K., Kenyon, S., Tuffnell, D. and Kurinczuk, J.J. (2020b) Characteristics and outcomes of pregnant women admitted to hospital with confirmed SARS-CoV-2 infection in UK: National population-based cohort study. *BMJ*, 369, m2107. Available at: https://doi.org/10.1136/bmj.m2107, accessed 12/06/2020.

Krieger, N. (1987) Shades of difference: theoretical underpinnings of the medical controversy on black/white differences in the United States, 1830–1870. *International Journal of Health Services*, 17(2), pp.259–78.

Kroll, M.E., Kurinczuk, J.J., Hollowell, J., Macfarlane, A., Li, Y. and Quigley, M. (2020) Ethnic and socioeconomic variation in cause-specific preterm infant mortality by gestational age at birth: national cohort study. *Archive of Disease in Childhood: Fetal and Neonatal Edition*, 105, pp.F56–F63.

Kumar, B.N. and Diaz, E. (2019) Migration health theories: Healthy migrant effect and allostatic load. Can both be true? *Migrant Health: A Primary Care Perspective*. Available at: https://doi.org/10.1201/9781351017190, accessed 02/04/2021.

Lacey, K.K., Park, J., Briggs, A.Q. and Jackson, J.S. (2019) National origins, social context, timing of migration and the physical and mental health of Caribbeans living in and outside of Canada. *Ethnicity & Health*, pp.1–24. Available at: https://doi.org/10.1080/13557858.2019.1634183, accessed 02/04/2021.

Lacobucci, G. (2020a) Covid-19: PHE review has failed ethnic minorities, leaders tell BMJ. *BMJ*, 369, m2264. Available at: https://doi.org/10.1136/bmj.m2264, accessed 12/06/2020.

Lacobucci, G. (2020b) Covid-19: Review of ethnic disparities is labelled 'whitewash' for lack of recommendations. *BMJ*, 369, m2208. Available at: doi:10.1136/bmj.m2208 pmid:32493696, accessed 12/06/2020.

Lamb, J., Bower, P., Rogers, A., Dowrick, C. and Gask, L. (2012) Access to mental health in primary care: A qualitative meta-synthesis of evidence from the experience of people from 'hard to reach' groups. *Health*, 16(1), pp.76–104.

LaPointe, L.L. (2012) *Paul Broca and the Origins of Language in the Brain*. San Diego: Plural Publishing.

Lawless, M.E., Muellner, J., Sehgal, A.R., Thomas, C.L. and Perzynski, A.T. (2014) Cultural competency education for researchers: A pilot study using a neighborhood visit approach. *SOCRA Source*, 81, pp.12–21.

Lawton, J., Ahmad, N., Hanna, L., Douglas, M. and Hallowell, N. (2006) 'I can't do any serious exercise': Barriers to physical activity among people of Pakistani and Indian origin with Type 2 diabetes. *Health Education Research*, 21(1), pp.43–54.

Lewis, G. (ed.) (2007) *The Confidential Enquiry into Maternal and Child Health (CEMACH). Saving Mothers' Lives: Reviewing maternal deaths to make motherhood safer – 2003–2005, The Seventh Report of Confidential Enquiries into Maternal Deaths in the United Kingdom.* London: CEMACH.

Lewis L., Taylor M., Broom J. and Johnston K.L. (2014) The cost-effectiveness of the Lighter Life weight management programme as an intervention for obesity in England. *Clinical Obesity*, 4(3), pp.180–188.

Likupe, G. and Archibong, U. (2013) Black African nurses' experiences of equality of opportunity, racism, and discrimination in the NHS. *Journal of Psychological Issues in Organizational Culture*, 3(S1), pp.227–246.

Liljas, A.E., Walters, K., Jovicic, A., Iliffe, S., Manthorpe, J., Goodman, C. and Kharicha, K. (2017) Strategies to improve engagement of 'hard to reach' older people in research on health promotion: A systematic review. *BMC Public Health*, 17(1), p.349.

Liljas, A.E., Walters, K., Jovicic, A., Iliffe, S., Manthorpe, J., Goodman, C. and Kharicha, K. (2019) Engaging 'hard to reach' groups in health promotion: The views of older people and professionals from a qualitative study in England. *BMC Public Health*, 19(1), pp.1–15.

Lincoln, Y. and Guba, E. (1985) *Naturalistic Inquiry Newbury Park.* London: Sage Publications.

Liu, J.J., Davidson, E., Bhopal, R.S., White, M., Johnson, M.R.D., Netto, G. and Sheikh, A. (2016) Adapting health promotion interventions for ethnic minority groups: A qualitative study. *Health Promotion International*, 31(2), pp.325–334.

Llácer, A., Zunzunegui, M.V., Del Amo, J., Mazarrasa, L. and Bolůmar, F. (2007) The contribution of a gender perspective to the understanding of migrants' health. *Journal of Epidemiology & Community Health*, 61(Suppl 2), pp.ii4-ii10.

Lombroso, C., Gibson, M. and Rafter, N.H. (2006) *Criminal Man.* Durham, NC: Duke University Press.

Malik, K. (1996) *The Meaning of Race: Race, history and culture in Western society.* Hampshire: Macmillan Press.

Malson, H. (2010) Qualitative methods from psychology, in I. Bourgeaul, R. Dingwall and R. De Vries (eds) *The SAGE Handbook Qualitative Methods Health Research.* London: Sage, pp.193–212.

Marmot, M. (2010) *Marmot Review. Fair Society, Healthy Lives: Strategic review of health inequalities in England post-2010.* London: The Marmot Review.

Marmot, M. (2020) Inequalities and Covid-19. *Royal Colleges of Physicians Commentary Magazine*, June, Issue 3. Available at: https://online.flowpaper.com/70b706f2/JuneCommentaryonline/#page=1, accessed 26/05/2020.

Marmot, M. and Allen, J. (2014) Social determinants of health equity. *American Journal of Public Health*, 104(S4), pp.S517-S519.

Marmot, M., Allen, J., Goldblatt, P., Herd, E. and Morrison, J. (2020) *Build Back Fairer: The COVID-19 Marmot Review, the pandemic, socioeconomic and health inequalities in England.* London: Institute of Health Equity.

Mason, D. (2000) *Race and Ethnicity in Modern Britain.* Oxford: Oxford University Press.

Mateos, P., Singleton, A. and Longley, P. (2009) Uncertainty in the analysis of ethnicity classifications: Issues of extent and aggregation of ethnic groups. *Journal of Ethnic and Migration Studies*, 35(9), pp.1437–1460.

Mathur, R., Hull, S.A., Badrick, E. and Robson, J. (2011) Cardiovascular multimorbidity: The effect of ethnicity on prevalence and risk factor management. *BJGP*, 61(586): pp.e262–70. doi: 10.3399/bjgp11X572454.

Maynard, M., Apekey, T.A., Kime, N., Walsh, D., Simpson, E. and Copeman, J. (2018) Views on risk, prevention and management of Type 2 diabetes among UK Black Caribbeans. *European Journal of Public Health*, 28(Suppl), p.99.

McAdams, D.P. (1988) *Power, Intimacy, and the Life Story: Personological inquiries into identity.* New York: Guilford Press.

McCabe, A., Gilchrist, A., Harris, K., Afridi, A. and Kyprianou, P. (2013) *Making the Links: Poverty, ethnicity and social networks.* York: Joseph Rowntree Foundation.

McGorrian, C., Hamid, N.A., Fitzpatrick, P., Daly, L., Malone, K.M. and Kelleher, C. (2013) Frequent mental distress (FMD) in Irish Travellers: Discrimination and bereavement negatively influence mental health in the All Ireland Traveller Health Study. *Transcultural Psychiatry*, 50(4), pp.559–578. doi:10.1177/1363461513503016.

McNabb, W., Quinn, M., Kerver, J., Cook, S. and Karrison, T. (1997) The PATHWAYS church-based weight loss program for urban African-American women at risk for diabetes. *Diabetes Care*, 20(10), pp.1518–1523.

Mead, G.H. (1934) *Mind, Self, and Society from the Standpoint of a Social Behaviorist*. Chicago: University of Chicago Press.

Mead, G.H. (2008) *The LSI*. Evanston, IL: The Foley Center for the Study of Lives, Northwestern University. Available at: http://www.sesp.northwestern.edu/foley/instruments/interview/, accessed 23/07/2020.

Memon, A., Taylor, K., Mohebati, L.M., Sundin, J., Cooper, M., Scanlon, T. and de Visser, R. (2016) Perceived barriers to accessing mental health services among black and minority ethnic (BME) communities: A qualitative study in Southeast England. *BMJ Open*, 6, e012337. doi:10.1136/bmjopen-2016-012337.

Millan, M. and Smith, D. (2019) A comparative sociology of Gypsy Traveller health in the UK. *International Journal of Environmental Research and Public Health*, 16(3), p.379.

Milner, A., Baker, E., Jeraj, S. and Butt, J. (2020) Race-ethnic and gender differences in representation within the English National Health Service: A quantitative analysis. *BMJ Open*, 10(2), e034258.

Miners, A., Harris, J., Felix, L., Murray, E., Michie, S. and Edwards, P. (2012) An economic evaluation of adaptive e-learning devices to promote weight loss via dietary change for people with obesity. *BMC Health Services Research*, 12, article 190. doi: 10.1186/1472-6963-12-190.

Mitchell, H.A., Allan, H. and Koch, T. (2017) Guyanese expatriate women ask: 'Is it a touch of sugar?'. *Action Research*, 18(4), pp.433–447. Available at: https://doi.org/10.1177/1476750317721303, accessed 08/08/2020

Moberly, T. (2018) Doctors from ethnic minority backgrounds earn less than white colleagues. *BMJ*, 363. Available at: doi:10.1136/bmj.k5089, accessed 02/04/2021.

Modood, T. (1994) Political blackness and British Asians. *Sociology*, 28(4), pp.859–876.

Møllersen, S. and Holte, A. (2008) Ethnicity as a variable in mental health research: A systematic review of articles published 1990–2004. *Nordic Journal of Psychiatry*, 62(4), pp.322–328.

Moore, A. (2020) Exclusive: Government censored BAME Covid-risk review. *Health Service Journal*. 3 June. Available at: https://www.hsj.co.uk/coronavirus/exclusive-government-censored-bame-covid-risk-review/7027761.article, accessed 15/06/2020.

Moore, A., Stanton-Fay, S., Rivas, C., Harding, S. and Goff, L. (2017) Co-design of a culturally-tailored diet & lifestyle intervention for diabetes management in the UK African-Caribbean community. *Proceedings of the Nutrition Society*, 76(OCE4), E163. Available at: https://doi:10.1017/S0029665117003251

Morgan, M. (1995) The significance of ethnicity for health promotion: patients' use of anti-hypertensive drugs in inner London. *International Journal of Epidemiology*, 24(Suppl. 1), pp.S79–S84.

Mori, D.L., Silberbogen, A.K., Collins, A.E., Ulloa, E.W., Brown, K.L. and Niles, B.L. (2011) Promoting physical activity in individuals with diabetes: Telehealth approaches. *Diabetes Spectrum*, 24(3), pp.127–135.

Morris, J. and O'Brien, E. (2011) Encouraging healthy outdoor activity among under-represented groups: An evaluation of the Active England woodland projects. *Urban Forestry & Urban Greening*, 10(4), pp.323–333.

Mukadam, N., Cooper, C., Basit, B. and Livingston, G. (2011) Why do ethnic elders present later to UK dementia services? A qualitative study. *International Psychogeriatrics*, 23(7), pp.1070–1077.

Mulholland, J. and Dyson, S. (2001) Sociological theories of 'race' and ethnicity, in ethnicity and nursing, in L. Practice, L. Culley and S. Dyson (eds) *Sociology and Nursing Practice*. Hampshire: Palgrave Macmillan, pp.17–38.

Mullings, L. and Schulz, A.J. (2006) Intersectionality and health: An introduction, in A.J. Schulz and L. Mullings (eds) *Gender, Race, Class, & Health: Intersectional approaches*. San Francisco, CA: Jossey-Bass, pp.3–17.

Mulugeta, B., Williamson, S., Monks, R., Hack, T. and Beaver, K. (2017) Cancer through black eyes: The views of UK based black men towards cancer: A constructivist grounded theory study. *European Journal of Oncology Nursing*, 29, pp.8–16.

Mwangi, E.W. and Constance-Huggins, M. (2017) Intersectionality and Black women's health: Making room for rurality. *Journal of Progressive Human Services*, 30(1), pp.11–24.

Narayan, J. (2019) British Black power: The anti-imperialism of political blackness and the problem of nativist socialism. *The Sociological Review*, 67(5), pp.945–967.

Nash, J.C. (2008) Re-thinking intersectionality. *Feminist Review*, 89(1), pp.1–15.

National Inclusion Health Board (NHIB) (2014) *Hidden Needs: Identifying key vulnerable groups in data collections*. Available at: https://assets. publishing.service.gov.uk/government/uploads/system/uploads/attachment_data/file/287805/vulnerable_groups_data_collections. pdf, accessed 15/06/200.

National Institute of Health Research (NIHR) (2020) *News: NIHR research ethnicity data provides insight on participation in Covid-19 studies*. Available at: https://www.nihr.ac.uk/news/nihr-research-ethnicity-data-provides-insight-on-participation-in-covid-19-studies/26460, accessed 22/12/20.

Nazroo, J.Y. (1997) *The Health of Britain's Ethnic Minorities: Findings from a national survey.* London: Policy Studies Institute.

Nazroo, J.Y., Bhui, K.S. and Rhodes, J. (2020) Where next for understanding race/ethnic inequalities in severe mental illness? Structural, interpersonal and institutional racism. *Sociology of Health & Illness,* 42(2), pp.262–276.

Nazroo J.Y., Falaschetti, E., Pierce, M. and Primatesta, P. (2009) Ethnic inequalities in access to and outcomes of healthcare: Analysis of the Health Survey for England. *Journal of Epidemiology and Community Health,* 63(12), pp.1022–1027.

Nazroo, N. (2003) The structuring of ethnic inequalities in health: Economic position, racial discrimination, and racism. *American Journal of Public Health,* 93(20), pp.277–284.

NHS Digital (2017) *Common Mental Disorders: Ethnicity and sex.* Available at: https://www.ethnicity-facts-figures.service.gov.uk/health/mental-health/adults-experiencing-common-mental-disorders/latest#full-page-history, accessed 23/06/2020.

NHS Digital (2018) *NHS Outcomes Framework: Inpatient satisfaction with hospital care.* Available at: https://www.ethnicity-facts-figures.service.gov.uk/health/patient-experience/inpatient-satisfaction-with-hospital-care/latest#by-ethnicity, accessed 01/06/2020.

NHS Digital (2019a) *National Child Measurement Programme England, 2016–17: Tables.* 2017. Available at: https://digital.nhs.uk/data-and-information/publications/statistical/national-child-measurement-programme/2016-17-school-year#resources, accessed 22/06/2020.

NHS Digital (2019b) *National Child Measurement Programme England, 2018-2019: Ethnicity.* Available at: https://digital.nhs.uk/data-and-information/publications/statistical/national-child-measurement-programme/2018-19-school-year/ethnicity, accessed 22/06/2020.

NHS Digital NHS Outcomes Framework (2019a) *Patient Experience of Primary Care: GP services.* Available at: https://www.ethnicity-facts-figures.service.gov.uk/health/patient-experience/patient-experience-of-primary-care-gp-services/latest#by-ethnicity, accessed 01/06/2020.

NHS Digital NHS Outcomes Framework (2019b) *Satisfaction with Access to GP Services.* Available at: https://www.ethnicity-facts-figures.service.gov.uk/health/patient-experience/satisfaction-with-access-to-gp-services/latest#by-ethnicity, accessed 01/06/2020.

NHS England (2014) *Five-year Forward View.* Available at: https://www.england.nhs.uk/wp-content/uploads/2014/10/5yfv-web.pdf, accessed 30/05/2020.

NHS England (2016) *Guide 07: Bite-size guide to diverse and inclusive participation.* Available at: https://www.england.nhs.uk/wp-content/uploads/2016/07/bitesize-guide-divers-inclusive.pdf, accessed 29/05/2020.

NHS England (2019) *Primary Medical Care Policy and Guidance Manual (PGM).* Available at: https://www.england.nhs.uk/publication/primary-medical-care-policy-and-guidance-manual-pgm/, accessed 10/05/2019.

NHS England (2020) *Supporting Pregnant Women Using Maternity Services During the Coronavirus Pandemic: Actions for NHS providers.* Version 1, 14 December. Available at: https://www.england.nhs.uk/coronavirus/wp-content/uploads/sites/52/2020/12/C0961-Supporting-pregnant-women-using-maternity-services-during-the-coronavirus-pandemic-actions-for-NHS-provi.pdf, accessed 22/12/2020.

NICE (2011) *Hypertension: Clinical management of primary hypertension in adults.* London: National Institute for Health and Clinical Excellence.

NICE (2013) *Public Health Guidance 46: Assessing body mass index and waist.* Available at: https://www.nice.org.uk/guidance/ph46, accessed 02/07/2020.

Niedzwiedz, C.L., O'Donnell, C.A., Jani, B.D., Demou, E., Ho, F.K., Celis-Morales, C., Nicholl, B.I., Mair, F.S., Welsh, P., Sattar, N. and Pell, J.P. (2020) Ethnic and socioeconomic differences in SARS-CoV-2 infection: Prospective cohort study using UK Biobank. *BMC Medicine*, 18(1), pp.1–14.

Noakes, H. (2010) Perceptions of black African and African-Caribbean people regarding insulin. *Journal of Diabetes Nursing*, 14(4), pp.148–155.

Nuffield Foundation (2020) *Covid-19 Social Study, Results Release 25.* Available at: https://mk0nuffieldfounpg9ee.kinstacdn.com/wp-content/uploads/2020/11/COVID-19-social-study-20-November-2020.pdf, accessed 22/12/2020.

O'Donnell, S. and Richardson, N. (2018) *Middle Aged Men and Suicide in Ireland: Men's Health Forum in Ireland.* Available at: http://www.mhfi.org/MAMRMreport.pdf, accessed 20/08/2020.

Office for National Statistics (ONS) (2011) *Census Data 2011.* Newport, UK: ONS.

Office for National Statistics (ONS) (2018) *Regional Ethnic Diversity, Census, 2011, Updated 1 August 2018.* Available at: https://www.ethnicity-facts-figures.service.gov.uk/british-population/national-and-regional-populations/regional-ethnic-diversity/latest, accessed 13/09/2018.

Office for National Statistics (ONS) (2019) *Ethnicity Pay Gaps in Great Britain: 2018*, 9 July, UK Government.

Office of Population, Censuses and Surveys (1995) *General Household Survey*. London: HMSO.

O'Mahony, J. (2017) *Traveller Community National Survey*. The Community Foundation for Ireland. Available at: http://www.communityfoundation.ie/images/uploads/pdfs/National-Traveller-Survey-2017.pdf, accessed 20/08/2020.

Papadopoulos, I. and Lees, S. (2002) Developing culturally competent researchers. *Journal of Advanced Nursing*, 37(3), pp.258–264.

Paul, S.K., Owusu Adjah, E.S., Samanta, M., Patel, K., Bellary, S., Hanif, W. and Khunti, K. (2017) Comparison of body mass index at diagnosis of diabetes in a multi-ethnic population: A case-control study with matched non-diabetic controls. *Diabetes, Obesity and Metabolism*, 19(7), pp.1014–1023.

Pearson, K. (1901) *Natural Life from the Standpoint of Science*. London: A&C Black.

Peplow, S. (2020) 'In 1997 nobody had heard of Windrush': The rise of the 'Windrush narrative' in British newspapers. *Immigrants & Minorities Historical Studies in Ethnicity, Migration and Diaspora*. Available at: https://doi.org/10.1080/02619288.2020.1781624, accessed 07/07/2020.

Phillips, T. and Phillips, M. (1998) *Windrush: The irresistible rise of multi-racial Britain*. London: Harper Collins.

Pickett, K.E. and Wilkinson, R.G. (2008) People like us: Ethnic group density effects on health. *Ethnicity & Health*, 13(4), pp.321–334.

Platt, L. (2007) *Poverty and Ethnicity in the UK* (vol. 2059). Joseph Rowntree Foundation. Bristol: Policy Press.

Pomerleau, J., McKeigue, P.M. and Chaturvedi, N. (1999) Factors associated with obesity in South Asian, Afro-Caribbean and European women. *International Journal of Obesity*, 23(1), pp.25–33.

Priest, N., Paradies, Y., Trenerry, B., Truong, M., Karlsen, S. and Kelly, Y. (2013) A systematic review of studies examining the relationship between reported racism and health and wellbeing for children and young people. *Social Science Medicine*, 95, pp.115–127.

Prinjha, S., Miah, N., Ali, E. and Farmer, A. (2020) Including 'seldom heard' views in research: Opportunities, challenges and recommendations from focus groups with British South Asian people with Type 2 diabetes. *BMC Medical Research Methodology*, 20(1), pp.1–11.

Public Health England (2016) *3.8 Million People in England Now Have Diabetes*. Available at: https://www.gov.uk/government/news/38-million-people-in-england-now-have-diabetes, accessed 17/01/2018.

Public Health England (2017) *Health and Wellbeing in Rural Areas*. Local Government Association. Available at: https://www.local.gov.uk/sites/default/files/documents/1.39_Health%20in%20rural%20areas_WEB.pdf, accessed 18/09/2018.

Public Health England (2018) *The Eatwell Guide*. Available at: https://assets.publishing.service.gov.uk/government/uploads/system/uploads/attachment_data/file/528193/Eatwell_guide_colour.pdf, accessed 30/09/2018.

Public Health England (2020a) *Disparities in the Risk and Outcomes of Covid-19*. June. Available at: https://assets.publishing.service.gov.uk/government/uploads/system/uploads/attachment_data/file/890258/disparities_review.pdf, accessed 12/06/2020.

Public Health England (2020b) *Beyond the Data: Understanding the impact of COVID-19 on BAME groups*. Available at: https://assets.publishing.service.gov.uk/government/uploads/system/uploads/attachment_data/file/892376/COVID_stakeholder_engagement_synthesis_beyond_the_data.pdf , accessed 24/06/2020.

Public Health England (2020c) *Rapid Investigation Team (RIT): Preliminary investigation into COVID-exceedances in Leicester* (June). Available at: https://assets.publishing.service.gov.uk/government/uploads/system/uploads/attachment_data/file/897128/COVID-19_activity_Leicester_Final-report_010720_v3.pdf, accessed 04/07/2020.

Qassem, T., Bebbington, P., Spiers, N., McManus, S., Jenkins, S. and Dein, S. (2015) Prevalence of psychosis in black ethnic minorities in Britain: Analysis based on three national surveys. *Social Psychiatry and Psychiatric Epidemiology*, 50(7), pp.1057–1064.

Race Disparity Unit (2019a) *Patient Experiences of Primary Care: GP services, ethnicity facts and figures*, 20 March, Gov.uk. Available at: https://www.ethnicity-facts-figures.service.gov.uk/health/patient-experiences/patient-experience-of-primary-care-gp-services/latest, accessed 19/09/2019.

Race Disparity Unit (2019b) *Health, Ethnicity, Facts and Figures*, 20 March, Gov.uk. Available at: https://www.ethnicity-facts-figures.service.gov.uk/health/patient-experiences/patient-experience-of-primary-care-gp-services/latest, accessed 19/09/2019.

Race Equality Foundation (2019) *Racial Disparities in Mental Health: Literature and evidence review.* Available at: https://raceequalityfoundation.org.uk/wp-content/uploads/2020/03/mental-health-report-v5-2.pdf, accessed 15/06/2020.

Rai, K.R. and Finch, H. (1997) *Physical Activity 'From our Point of View': Qualitative research among South Asian and Black communities.* London: Health Education Authority UK.

Raisi-Estabragh, Z., McCracken, C., Bethell, M., Cooper, J., Cooper, C., Caulfield, M., Munroe, P., Harvey, N. and Petersen, S. (2020) Greater risk of severe COVID-19 in Black, Asian and Minority Ethnic populations is not explained by cardiometabolic, socioeconomic or behavioural factors, or by 25 (OH)-vitamin D status: Study of 1326 cases from the UK Biobank. *Journal of Public Health*, 42(3), pp.451–460.

Ray, L. and Reed, K. (2005) Community, mobility and racism in a semi-rural area: Comparing minority experience in East Kent. *Ethnic and Racial Studies*, 28(2), pp.212–234.

Razieh, C., Khunti, K., Davies, M., Edwardson, C., Henson, J., Darko, N., Comber, A., Jones, A. and Yates, T. (2019) Association of depression and anxiety with clinical, sociodemographic, lifestyle and environmental factors in South Asian and white European people at high risk of diabetes. *Diabetic Medicine.* doi: 10.1111/dme.13986.

RE-AIM.org (2018) *What is REAIM.* Available at: http://www.re-aim.org, accessed 10/09/2018.

Reimer-Kirkham, S. and Sharma, S. (2011) Adding religion to gender, race, and class: Seeking new insights on intersectionality in health care contexts, in O. Hankivsky (ed.) *Health Inequities in Canada: Intersectional frameworks and practices.* Vancouver, Canada: University of British Columbia Press, pp.112–131.

Rimmer, J.H., Rubin, S.S. and Braddock, D. (2000) Barriers to exercise in African American women with physical disabilities. *Archives of Physical Medicine and Rehabilitation*, 81(2), pp.182–188.

Riste, L., Khan, F. and Cruickshank, K. (2001) High prevalence of Type 2 diabetes in all ethnic groups, including Europeans, in a British inner city: Relative poverty, history, inactivity, or 21st century Europe? *Diabetes Care*, 24(8), pp.1377–1383.

Rivenbark, J.G. and Ichou, M. (2020) Discrimination in healthcare as a barrier to care: Experiences of socially disadvantaged populations in France from a nationally representative survey. *BMC Public Health*, 20(1), p.31.

Rizzolo, K., Jaber, M., Schaumburg, J., Vakil-Gilani, K. and Rebusi, N. (2020) *Evaluation of a Resident-Driven Trauma-Sensitive Yoga Program for Female Immigrant Primary Care Patients*, Costas T. Lambrew Research Retreat 2020. 62. Available at: https://knowledgeconnection. mainehealth.org/lambrew-retreat-2020/62, accessed 20/08/2020.

Roberts, B. (2001) *Biographical Research*. Buckingham: Open University Press.

Rockliffe, L., Chorley, A.J., Marlow, L.A. and Forster, A.S. (2018) It's hard to reach the 'hard-to-reach': The challenges of recruiting people who do not access preventative healthcare services into interview studies. *International Journal of Qualitative Studies on Health and Well-Being*, 13(1). DOI: 10.1080/17482631.2018.1479582

Rowe, N. and Chapman, R. (2000) *Sports Participation and Ethnicity in England. National Survey 1999/2000: Headline findings.* London: Sport England.

Salisbury, C., Johnson, L., Purdy, S., Valderas, J.M. and Montgomery, A.A. (2011) Epidemiology and impact of multimorbidity in primary care: A retrospective cohort study. *BJGP*, 61(582), pp.e12–21. doi: 10.3399/bjgp11X548929.

Salway, S., Mir, G., Turner, D., Ellison, G.T., Carter, L. and Gerrish, K. (2016) Obstacles to 'race equality' in the English National Health Service: Insights from the healthcare commissioning arena. *Social Science & Medicine*, 152, pp.102–110.

Sands, S.R., Ingraham, K. and Salami, B.O. (2020) Caribbean nurse migration: A scoping review. *Human Resources for Health*, 18(1), pp.1–10.

Sargeant, J.A., Yates, T., McCann, G.P., Lawson, C.A., Davies, M.J., Gulsin, G.S. and Henson, J. (2018) Physical activity and structured exercise in patients with Type 2 diabetes mellitus and heart failure. *Practical Diabetes*, 35(4), pp.131–138b.

Saunders, C.L., Abel, G.A., El Turabi, A., Ahmed, F. and Lyratzopoulos, G. (2013) Accuracy of routinely recorded ethnic group information compared with self-reported ethnicity: Evidence from the English Cancer Patient Experience survey. *BMJ Open*, 3(6), e002882. doi: 10.1136/bmjopen-2013-002882.

Saxena, S., Ambler, G., Cole, T.J. and Majeed, A. (2004) Ethnic group differences in overweight and obese children and young people in England: Cross sectional survey. *Archives of Disease in Childhood*, 89(1), pp.30–36.

Schwingel, A., Gálvez, P., Linares, D. and Sebastião, E. (2017) Using a mixed-methods RE-AIM framework to evaluate community health programs for older Latinas. *Journal of Aging and Health*, 29(4), pp.551–593.

Scott, P. (2001) Caribbean people's health beliefs about the body and their implications for diabetes management: A South London study. *Practical Diabetes International*, 18(3), pp.94–98.

Semlyen, J., Ali, A. and Flowers, P. (2018) Intersectional identities and dilemmas in interactions with healthcare professionals: An interpretative phenomenological analysis of British Muslim gay men. *Culture, Health & Sexuality*, 20(9), pp.1023–1035.

Sengupta, P. (2012) Health impacts of yoga and pranayama: A state-of-the-art review. *International Journal of Preventive Medicine*, 3(7), pp.444–458.

Shaghaghi, A., Bhopal, R.S. and Sheikh, A. (2011) Approaches to recruiting 'hard-to-reach' populations into research: A review of the literature. *Health Promotion Perspectives*, 1(2), pp.86–94.

Shah, M., Radia, D. and McCarthy, H.D. (2020) Waist circumference centiles for UK South Asian children. *Archives of Disease in Childhood*, 105(1), pp.80–85.

Shaw, N.J., Crabtree, N.J., Kibirige, M.S. and Fordham, J. (2007) Ethnic and gender differences in body fat in British schoolchildren as measured by DXA. *Archives of Disease in Childhood*, 92(10), pp.872–875.

Sheldon, T.A. and Parker, H. (1992) Race and ethnicity in health research. *Journal of Public Health*, 14(2), pp.104–110.

Shoneye, C., Johnson, F., Steptoe, A. and Wardle, J. (2011) A qualitative analysis of black and white British women's attitudes to weight and weight control. *Journal of Human Nutrition and Dietetics*, 24(6), pp.536–542.

Smith, K.E., Bambra, C. and Hill, S.E. (2016) Background and introduction: UK experiences of health inequalities, in K.E. Smith, C. Bambra and S.E. Hill (eds) *Health Inequalities: Critical perspectives*. Oxford: Oxford University Press.

Smith, P. and Mackintosh, M. (2007) Profession, market and class: Nurse migration and the remaking of division and disadvantage. *Journal of Clinical Nursing*, 16(12), pp.2213–2220.

Sproston, K. and Mindell, J. (2006) *Health Survey for England 2004 Vol 1&2: The health of minority ethnic groups*. London: The Information Centre. Available at: https://files.digital.nhs.uk/publicationimport/pub01xxx/pub01170/hea-surv-ethn-min-eng-2004-rep-v3.pdf, accessed 29/08/2020.

Strauss, A. and Corbin, J. (1998) *Basics of Qualitative Research: Procedures and techniques for developing grounded theory*. London: Sage.

Stronks, K. and Kunst, A.E. (2009) The complex interrelationship between ethnic and socio-economic inequalities in health. *Journal of Public Health*, 31(3), pp.324–325.

Sutaria, S., Mathur, R. and Hull, S.A. (2019) Does the ethnic density effect extend to obesity? A cross-sectional study of 415 166 adults in east London. *BMJ Open*, 9(5), e024779.

Sutherland, M.E. (2006) African Caribbean immigrants in the United Kingdom: The legacy of racial disadvantages. *Caribbean Quarterly*, 52(1), pp.26–52. Available at: www.jstor.org/stable/40654533, accessed 19/07/2020.

Sydor, A. (2013) Conducting research into hidden or hard-to-reach populations. *Nurse Researcher*, 20(3), pp.33–37. https://doi.org/10.7748/ nr2013.01.20.3.33.c9495.

Szczepura, A. (2005) Access to health care for ethnic minority populations. *Postgraduate Medical Journal*, 81(953), pp.141–147.

Taylor, C.M. (1981) W.E.B. DuBois's challenge to scientific racism, *Journal of Black Studies*, 11(4), pp.449–460.

Taylor, R. (2018) *Impact of 'Hostile Environment' Policy*, Debate on 14 June 2018. House of Lords Library Briefing.

Tenfelde, S.M., Hatchett, L. and Saban, K.L. (2018) 'Maybe black girls do yoga': A focus group study with predominantly low-income African American women. *Complementary Therapies in Medicine*, 40, pp.230–235.

The Guardian (2020) Calls mount for public inquiry into UK BAME Covid-19 death rate, 2 June. Available at: https://www.theguardian.com/world/2020/jun/02/calls-mount-for-public-inquiry-into-uk-bame-covid-19-death-rate, accessed 15/06/2020.

Thompson, N. (2013) *Leeds Gypsy and Traveller Community Health Needs Assessment*. LeedsGate: Leeds Gypsy and Traveller Exchange.

Thorogood, N. (1989) Afro-Caribbean women's experience of the health service. *Journal of Ethnic and Migration Studies*, 15(3), pp.319–334.

Tillin, T., Forouhi, N.G., McKeigue, P.M. and Chaturvedi, N. (2010) Southall and Brent revisited: Cohort profile of SABRE, a UK population-based comparison of cardiovascular disease and diabetes in people of European, Indian Asian and African Caribbean origins. *International Journal of Epidemiology*, 41(1), pp.33–42.

Tillin, T., Hughes, D., Godsland, I., Whincup, P., Forouhi, N., Welsh, P., Sattar, N., McKeigue, P. and Chaturvedi, N. (2013) Insulin resistance and truncal obesity as important determinants of the greater incidence of diabetes in Indian Asians and African Caribbeans compared with Europeans. *Diabetes Care*, 36(2), pp.383–393. DOI: 10.2337/dc12-0544.

Tolley, E.E., Ulin, P.R., Mack, N., Robinson, E.T. and Succop, S.M. (2016) *Qualitative Methods in Public Health: A field guide for applied research*, 2nd edn. San Francisco: John Wiley & Sons.

Tomalin, E., Sadgrove, J. and Summers, R. (2019) Health, faith and therapeutic landscapes: Places of worship as Black, Asian and Minority Ethnic (BAME) public health settings in the United Kingdom. *Social Science & Medicine*, 230, pp.57–65.

Toobert, D.J., Strycker, L.A., Glasgow, R.E. and Bagdade, J.D. (2002) If you build it, will they come? Reach and adoption associated with a comprehensive lifestyle management program for women with Type 2 diabetes. *Patient Education and Counselling*, 48(2), pp.99–105.

Townsend, P. (2017) *UK Townsend Deprivation Scores*. Available at: https://www.statistics.digitalresources.jisc.ac.uk/dataset/2011-uk-townsend-deprivation-scores, accessed 29/06/2020.

Tran, V.D., Do, V.V., Pham, N.M., Nguyen, C.T., Xuong, N.T., Jancey, J. and Lee, A.H. (2020) Validity of the international physical activity questionnaire – short form for application in Asian countries: A study in Vietnam. *Evaluation & the Health Professions*, 43(2), pp.105–109.

Tritter, J. and Lester, H. (2007) Health inequalities and user involvement, in E. Dowler and N. Spencer (eds) *Challenging Health Inequalities: Multi-disciplinary perspectives*. Bristol: Policy Press, pp.175–192.

Truswell, D. (2019) Dementia and the UK African-Caribbean community, in D. Truswell (ed) *Supporting People Living with Dementia in Black, Asian and Minority Ethnic Communities: Key issues and strategies for change*. London: Jessica Kingsley, pp.35–54.

Turner, L.W., Sutherland, M., Harris, G., Barber, M. (1995) Cardiovascular health promotion in north Florida African American churches. *Health Values*, 19(2), pp.3–9.

Two Feathers, J., Kieffer, E.C., Palmisano, G., Anderson, M., Sinco, B., Janz, N., Heisler, M., Spencer, M., Guzman, R., Thompson, J. and Wisdom, K. (2005) Racial and Ethnic Approaches to Community Health (REACH) Detroit partnership: Improving diabetes-related outcomes among African American and Latino adults. *American Journal of Public Health*, 95(9), pp.1552–1560.

Van Den Berghe, P.L. (1981) *The Ethnic Phenomenon*. New York: Elsevier.

Van Evera, S. (2001) 'Primordialism lives!' *APSA-CP: Newsletter of the Organized Section in Comparative Politics of the American Political Science Association,* 12(1), pp.20–22.

Visram, S., Crosland, A., Unsworth, J. and Long, S. (2007) Engaging women from South Asian communities in cardiac rehabilitation. *British Journal of Community Nursing,* 12(1), pp.13–18.

Walker, S. (2020) Systemic Racism: Big, black, mad and dangerous in the criminal justice system, in R. Majors, K. Carberry and T.S. Ranshaw (eds) *The International Handbook of Black Community Mental Health.* Bingley: Emerald Publishing Limited, pp.41–60.

Wallace, S., Nazroo, J.Y. and Bécares, L. (2016) Cumulative effect of racial discrimination on the mental health of ethnic minorities in the United Kingdom. *American Journal of Public Health,* 106(7), pp.1294–1300.

Walsh, D.C., Rudd, R.E., Moeykens, B.A. and Moloney, T. (1993) Social marketing for public health. *Health Affairs,* 12(2), pp.104–119.

Watkins, D.C., Walker, R.L. and Griffith, D.M. (2010) A meta-study of Black male mental health and well-being. *Journal of Black Psychology,* 36(3), pp.303–330.

Watson, N. (2013) Exploring the role of support in the lived experiences of Black British African Caribbean nurses as students and staff in the British NHS. *Blackness in Britain,* 12 September, Newman University, Birmingham.

Weller, S.J., Crosby, L.J., Turnbull, E.R., Burns, R., Miller, A., Jones, L. and Aldridge, R.W. (2019) The negative health effects of hostile environment policies on migrants: A cross-sectional service evaluation of humanitarian healthcare provision in the UK. *Wellcome Open Research,* 172(109), pp.1–14.

WHO (2004) *Poverty: Assessing the distribution of health risks by socioeconomic position at national and local levels.* Environmental burden of disease series No. 10. Geneva: World Health Organization. Available at: https://www.who.int/quantifying_ehimpacts/publications/ebd10.pdf?ua=1, accessed 24/06/2020.

Williams, D.R. (1994) The concept of race in health services research: 1966 to 1990. *Health Services Research,* 29(3), pp.261–274.

Williams, D.R. and Mohammed, S.A. (2009) Discrimination and racial disparities in health: Evidence and needed research. *Journal of Behavioral Medicine,* 32(1), pp.20–47.

Williams, D.R., Lawrence, J.A. and Davis, B.A. (2019) Racism and health: Evidence and needed research. *Annual Review of Public Health,* 40, pp.105–125.

Wittkowski, A., Zumla, A., Glendenning, S. and Fox J.R.E. (2011) The experience of postnatal depression in South Asian mothers living in Great Britain: A qualitative study. *Reproductive and Infant Psychology*, 29(5), pp.480–492.

Wolf, R.M., Nagpal, M. and Magge, S.N. (2020) Diabetes and cardiometabolic risk in South Asian youth: A review. *Pediatric Diabetes*, 22(1), pp.52–66.

Wolfe, C.D.A., Rudd, A.G., Howard, R., Coshall, C., Stewart, J., Lawrence, E., Hajat, C. and Hillen, T. (2002) Incidence and case fatality rates of stroke subtypes in a multiethnic population: The South London Stroke Register. *Journal of Neurology, Neurosurgery & Psychiatry*, 72(2), pp.211–216.

Wozniak, L., Soprovich, A., Mundt, C., Johnson, J.A. and Johnson, S.T. (2015) Contextualizing the proven effectiveness of a lifestyle intervention for Type 2 diabetes in primary care: A qualitative assessment based on the RE-AIM Framework. *Canadian Journal of Diabetes*, 39(3), pp.S92–9.

Wray, S. and Bartholomew, M.L. (2006) Older African Caribbean women: The influence of migration on experiences of health and well-being in later life. *Research Policy and Planning*, 24(2), pp.103–119.

Yanek, L.R., Becker, D.M., Moy, T.F., Gittelsohn, J. and Koffman, D.M. (2016) Project Joy: Faith based cardiovascular health promotion for African American women. *Public Health Reports*, 116(Suppl 1), pp.68–81.

Yin, R.K. (2009) *Case Study Research, Design and Method*. London: Sage.

Young, D.R. and Stewart, K.J. (2006) A church-based physical activity intervention for African American women. *Family & Community Health*, 29(2), pp.103–117.

Index

Note: Page numbers in **bold** indicate tables.

A

age 80–1
anti-racist movement 11
anxiety
 black African-Caribbeans 118, 134
 BME groups 26
 BME women 27, 96
 Gypsies, Roma and Travellers 25
 South Asian women 95, 96, 98
Asian women
 maternal mortality 32
 maternity care 36
 see also South Asian women
Asians 27, 40
 see also South Asians

B

Bangladeshis
 COVID-19 27
 health inequalities 20, 21
 income inequality 33
 lifestyle behaviour change
  interventions 62
 obesity 23, 24
 patient experience 35–6
biological determinism 6, 7
Black, Asian and Minority Ethnic
 (BAME) 5, 6, 10, 11, 12–13, 26
black adults 23
black African American men 48, 49
black African American women 58
black African Americans 2, 7, 8, 41
black African-Caribbeans
 ethnic health inequalities 20, 21
 cardiovascular disease 22
 COVID-19 27
 infant mortality 32
 mental health conditions 24–5, 26
 obesity 24
 patient experience 35
 Type 2 diabetes mellitus
  (T2DM) 23, 54–5
 ethnicity recording 41
 health and wellbeing 110–36
 life story interview guide **116**
 life story interviews 115–33
 life story method 112–14, 136–7
 hostile environment policy 108–10
 UK population 107
 'Windrush generation' 108

 see also British African-
  Caribbean women
black Africans
 cardiovascular disease 22, 23
 ethnicity recording 41
 health inequalities 20, 21
 income inequality 32
 mental health conditions 24–5
 obesity 24
Black and Minority Ethnic (BME) 5,
 6, 10, 11–13, 19, 137
 'hard to reach' 14–16, 112
Black and Minority Ethnic (BME)
 migrant women
 physical activity programme 93–106
 aims and objectives 96–7
 limitations and
  recommendations 103–5
 programme evaluation 97–103
 project and background 93–6
black men 26
 see also black African American men
black women
 COVID-19 27
 intersectionality 47
 maternal mortality 32, 36
 maternity care 36
 see also black African American
  women; Black and Minority Ethnic
  (BME) migrant women; British
  African-Caribbean woman
Body Mass Index (BMI) 24, 81
British African-Caribbean
 women 53–91
 'hard to reach' 55–6
 intersectionality 58–60
 lifestyle behaviour change
  interventions 56–7
 programme assessment 63–91
 programme description 60–3
 research methods 60
 Type 2 diabetes mellitus
  (T2DM) 53–5
Broca, Paul 6

C

cancer 20, 21
cardiovascular disease 20, 21, 27,
 94, 110
 health-related risk factors 22–4, 32

care responsibilities 83–4
change, need for 132–3, 135
Chicago School 113
childcare 102, 105
children 20, 23–4
Chinese men 23
Chinese people 27, 33, 35, 40
chronic health conditions
  African-Caribbean migrants 110,
    118, 120, 134
  BME groups 27
  South Asians 94
churches 88
community champions 90
co-morbidities 27, 28
constructivism 6, 9, 10, 60, 77, 114
COVID-19 2, 11, 26–9
  black African-Caribbeans 115, 130–2
  BME NHS staff 35
  and deprivation 32
COVID-19 studies 39–40
COVID-19 tests 13
Crenshaw, Kimberlé 46, 59
critical life episodes 115
cultural competency 43

D

dance classes 86
Darwin, Charles 6
  see also social Darwinism
data *see* ethnic health data
Department of Health 13
depression 25, 27, 95, 96, 111
deprivation 31, 32, 94, 103
diabetes 20
  see also Type 2 diabetes mellitus
  (T2DM)
digital interventions 88–9
disability 80–1
discrimination 16, 17, 34–6, 110, 126,
  134, 137
domestic violence *see* partner violence
Du Bois, W.E.B. 7–8

E

Eatwell Plate 61, 85
employment 119–20, 125, 126–8
employment type 33–4
epistemology 113
Equality Act 2010 11, 12, 16, 30, 42
Equality Act 2020 16
ethnic health data 37
  data recording 39–42, 56, 138, 139
  ethnicity and race concepts 37–9
  health research 42–3
ethnic health inequalities 19–22
  cardiovascular disease 22–4

COVID-19 26–9, 32
  intersectionality 47
  mental health conditions 24–6
  social, cultural and economic
    factors 29–31
  socioeconomic status 31–4
  structural racism and discrimination
    34–6
ethnic minorities 10, 11
ethnic minority groups 13, 19, 137
  'hard to reach' 14–16
  infant mortality 32
ethnicity 6, 8–11, 12, 37–9, 137
  see also race
ethnicity recording 39–42, 56,
  138, 139
eugenics 7

F

faith 59, 88
family 83–4
Floyd, George 2

G

Gabriel, R.H. 7
Galton, Francis 7
gay men 50–1
gender 20, 23, 27–8, 46, 48–9, 83
geographical location 59, 82
'good health' 118, 119
'good mental health' 118, 134
GP services 35
Gypsies 12
  ethnicity recording 41
  health inequalities 20, 21
  mental health conditions 25
  patient experience 35

H

Hancock, Matt 2
'hard to reach' 1, 2, 5, 13–16, 137, 138
  black African-Caribbeans 130, 135
  BME groups 112
  BME migrant women 95
  British African-Caribbean
    women 53, 55–6, 59, 79–80, 84, 90
health data *see* ethnic health data
health inequalities *see* ethnic
  health inequalities
health promotion 49
health research 42–3, 138, 139
healthcare professionals 126–8
'Healthier You' programme 88–9
health-related risk factors 21–2
  cardiovascular disease 22–4, 32
healthy eating 49, 60, 61–2, 84–6, 97
Hitler, Adolf 7

HIV prevention 49
homogeneity 15–16, 80
Hong King 50
hope 132–3, 135
hospital services 35–6

I

immigration *see* migration
Immigration Act 1972 109
income inequality 32–4
Indians 22, 23, 27, 35
infant mortality 21, 32
institutional racism 34, 127
instrumentalism 9
interpretivism 113
intersectionality 80–1, 133, 135, 138
intersectionality framework 70
intersectionality theory 45–8
   lifestyle behaviour change
      interventions 58–60, 61
   preventative health and lifestyle
      interventions 48–51
intimate relationships 50
Irish people 21
Irish Travellers 20, 21, 35, 41

J

Jensen, Arthur 7
Johnson, M.R.D. 9, 12

K

keyworkers 33
Kidd, Benjamin 7
kidney disease 22

L

life story interview guide **116**
life story interviews
   data collection 115–18
   findings and discussion 118–33
life story method 112–14, 136–7
lifestyle behaviour change
      interventions 56–7
   intersectionality 58–60
   programme assessment 63–91
      data analysis 69–77
      interview guide **66–8**
      research questions 65, 69
      results and discussion 77–90
   programme description 60–3
Lombroso, Cesare 6

M

Marmot Review 30
masculinity 48–9
maternal mortality 32, 36
maternity care 36

May, Theresa 108
McAdams, D.P. 115
mental health 102
   'good mental health' 118, 134
mental health conditions 20, 24–6, 111
mental health interventions 50
mental health support 122–3
migrant status
   and hostile environment
      policy 108–10
   impact on health and
      wellbeing 110–12
   life story interview guide **116**
   life story interviews 115–33
migrant women *see* Black and Minority
   Ethnic (BME) migrant women
migration 107, 108
modernism 9
mortality 95
   infant mortality 21, 32
   maternal mortality 32, 36
Muslim gay men 50–1
Muslim women 94, 100

N

National Health Service (NHS)
   ethnicity monitoring 10, 41, 56
   'hard to reach' 13
NHS staff 33, 35
   discrimination 126–8, 131
nurses 126–8

O

obesity 20, 21, 22
   black African American men 48
   BME migrant women 95
   British African-Caribbean women 55
   children 23–4
   and racial isolation 81
   South Asian women 94, 98
ontology 113–14
othering 1, 5, 14, 56

P

Pakistanis
   cardiovascular disease 22
   COVID-19 26, 27
   health inequalities 20, 21, 32
   health promotion 49
   income inequality 33
   obesity 24
   patient experience 35
partner violence 50
patient experience 35–6
pay gap 32–4
Pearson, Karl 7
perennialism 9

physical activity 61, 62, 85, 86
physical activity programme 93–106
  aims and objectives 96–7
  limitations and
    recommendations 103–5
  programme evaluation 97–103
  project and background 93–6
physical inactivity 23, 48, 55, 94
police brutality 2
political blackness 11
positivism 113
pregnant women 27–8
preventative health and lifestyle
    interventions 48–51
primordialism 8–9
prostate cancer 21
psychosis 26
psychotic disorders 21, 35

R

race 6–8, 10, 11, 16, 37–9, 46,
    137
  see also ethnicity
racial discrimination see discrimination
racial stereotyping 26, 36, 128–
    30, 134–5
racism 78, 84, 110, 111, 121, 126
  institutional 34, 127
  scientific 6–7
  structural 34–5, 119, 124, 125,
    131, 134
RE-AIM assessment tool 63–77
  data analysis 69–77
  interview guide **66–8**
  research questions 65, 69
realism 114
reflexivity 77
relationships 50
  see also partner violence
religion 48, 50, 59, 88, 94, 100
Roma 12, 25, 41
rural areas 59, 80–1

S

Samoa 50
scientific racism 6–7
sexual minorities 50–1
skin colour 6
Soca sessions 86
social constructivism see constructivism
social Darwinism 7
social determinants of health see wider
    social determinants of health
social isolation 59, 80–2, 94–5, 96,
    102–3, 104, 106
social media 105
socioeconomic factors 57

socioeconomic positioning 82–3, 83–4
socioeconomic status 31–4, 59, 80–1
South Asian children 23–4
South Asian men 55
South Asian women
  maternity care 36
  mental disorders 25
  physical activity programme 93–106
    aims and objectives 96–7
    limitations and
      recommendations 103–5
    programme evaluation 97–103
    project and background 93–6
South Asians
  cardiovascular disease 22, 94
  chronic health conditions 94
  COVID-19 26
  lifestyle behaviour change
    interventions 61–2
  programme assessment 64
stress 25, 95, 118, 134
stroke 22, 110
structural racism 34–5, 119, 124, 125,
    131, 134
suicide 25
symbolic interactionism 114

T

trauma 121–5, 134
Travellers 12, 20, 21, 25, 35, 41
Type 2 diabetes mellitus (T2DM)
    22–3, 53–4
  lifestyle behaviour change
    interventions 56–7
  and intersectionality 58–60
  programme assessment 63–91
  programme description 60–3
  research methods 60
  risk and prevalence in BME
    groups 54–5
  South Asian women 98
  South Asians 94

U

'underserved groups' 14
unemployment 57
urban locations 59

W

West Indies 107, 108
WhatsApp 105
white minorities 12, 41
wider social determinants of health
    28–9, 30–1, 48–9
  socioeconomic status 31–4
'Windrush generation' 108
  health and wellbeing 111

hostile environment policy 109–10, 135
life story interviews 117, 118, 121, 123, 125–6
'Windrush scandal' 109–10
women-only physical activity programme 93–106
aims and objectives 96–7
limitations and recommendations 103–5
programme evaluation 97–103
project and background 93–6

work patterns 57, 82, 87, 120

Y

yoga programme 93–106
aims and objectives 96–7
limitations and recommendations 103–5
programme evaluation 97–103
project and background 93–6
yoga sessions 62, 86, 87
young people 50